A FEAST OF INFORMATION—

for people who love to eat but need to know the carbohydrate count of their meals.

THE BARBARA KRAUS 1980 CARBOHYDRATE GUIDE TO BRAND NAMES & BASIC FOODS lists thousands of basic and ready-to-eat foods from appetizers to desserts—carry it to the supermarket, to the restaurant, to the beach, to the coffee cart, and on trips.

Flip through these fact-filled pages. Mix, match, and keep track of grams as they add up. But remember, strawberry shortcake is fattening any way you slice it!

THE BARBARA KRAUS 1980 CARBOHYDRATE GUIDE TO BRAND NAMES & BASIC FOODS

The Barbara Kraus 1980 Carbohydrate Guide to Brand Names and Basic Foods

A SIGNET BOOK

NEW AMERICAN LIBRARY

TIMES MIRROR

For Bernice, Michael and James Molina

Excerpted from *Dictionary of Calories and Carbohydrates*

Foreword

The composition of the foods we eat is not static: it changes from time to time. In the case of *brand-name* products, manufacturers alter their recipes to reflect the availability of ingredients, advances in technology, or improvements in formulae. Each year new products appear on the market and some old ones are discontinued.

On the other hand, information on *basic foods* such as meats, vegetables, and fruits may also change as a result of the development of better analytical methods, different growing conditions, or new marketing practices. These changes, however, are usually relatively small as compared with those in manufactured products.

Some differences may be found between the values in this book and those appearing on the product labels. This is usually due to the fact that the Food and Drug Administration permits manufacturers to round the figures reported on labels. The data in this book are reported as calculated without rounding. If large differences between the two sets of values are noted, they may be due to changes in product formulae, and in those cases the label data should be used.

For all these reasons, a book of carbohydrate or nutritive values of foods must be kept up to date by a periodic reviewing and revision of the data presented.

Therefore, this handy carbohydrate counter will provide each year the most current and accurate estimates available. Generous use of this little book will help you and your family to select the right foods and the proper number of carbohydrates each member requires.

Good eating in 1980! For 1981, we'll pick up the new products, drop any has-beens, and make whatever other changes are necessary.

Barbara Kraus

Why This Book?

Some of the data presented here can be found in more detail in my best-selling *Calories and Carbohydrates,* a dictionary of 8,000 brand names and basic foods. Complete as it is, it is meant to be used as a reference book at home or in the office and not to be squeezed into a suit jacket or evening bag—it's just too big.

Therefore, responding to the need for a portable carbohydrate guide, and one which can reflect food changes often, I have written this smaller and handier version. The selection of material and the additional new entries provide the reader with pertinent data on thousands of products that they would prepare at home to take to work, eat in a restaurant or luncheonette, nibble on from the coffee cart, take to the beach, buy in the candy store, etcetera.

For the sake of saving space and providing you with a greater selection of products, I had to make certain compromises: whereas in the giant book there are several physical descriptions of a product, here there is but one; and when there is only one-tenth gram carbohydrate variance between brands, both products will bear the same number, since such variances are not only unimportant in dieting, but are also often due only to a different way of rounding numbers.

What Are Carbohydrates?

Carbohydrates—which include sugars, starches, and acids —are one of several chemical compounds in food which yield calories. Their main function is to supply energy to body cells, particularly muscle and brain cells. The amount of carbohydrates varies from zero in meats, fish, and poultry, to heavy concentrations in such foods as syrups, cereals, bread, beans, some fresh and all dried fruit, and root vegetables, such as potatoes.

As of this date, the most respected nutritional researchers insist that some carbohydrate is necessary every day for maintaining good health. The amount to be included is an individual matter, and in any drastic effort to alter your eating patterns, be sure to consult your doctor first.

ABBREVIATIONS AND SYMBOLS

* = prepared as package directs[1]
< = less than
& = and
" = inch
canned = bottles or jars as well as cans
dia. = diameter
fl. = fluid
liq. = liquid
lb. = pound
med. = medium

oz. = ounce
pkg. = package
pt. = pint
qt. =quart
sq. = square
T. = tablespoon
Tr. = trace
tsp. = teaspoon
wt. = weight

Italics or name in parentheses = registered trademark, ®. All data not identified by company or trademark are based on material obtained from the United States Department of Agriculture or Health, Education and Welfare/Food and Agriculture Organization.

EQUIVALENTS

By Weight	By Volume
1 pound = 16 ounces	1 quart = 4 cups
1 ounce = 28.35 grams	1 cup = 8 fluid ounces
3.52 ounces = 100 grams	1 cup = ½ pint
	1 cup = 16 tablespoons
	2 tablespoons = 1 fluid ounce
	1 tablespoon = 3 teaspoons
	1 pound butter = 4 sticks or 2 cups

---

[1] If the package directions call for whole or skim milk, the data given here are for whole milk unless otherwise stated.

Food and Description	Measure or Quantity	Carbohydrates (grams)

A

AC'CENT	¼ tsp.	0
ALEXANDER COCKTAIL MIX		
(Holland House)	1 serving	16.0
ALLSPICE (French's)	1 tsp.	1.3
ALMOND:		
In shell	10 nuts	2.0
Shelled, raw, natural, with skins	1 oz.	5.5
Roasted, dry (Planters)	1 oz.	6.0
ALPHA-BITS (Post)	1 cup	23.8
A.M. FRUIT DRINK		
(Mott's)	6 fl. oz.	22.0
ANCHOVY, PICKLED	2-oz. can	.1
APPLE:		
Eaten with skin	2½″ dia.	15.3
Eaten without skin	2½″ dia.	13.9
Dried (Del Monte)	1 cup	37.2
Frozen, sweetened	10-oz. pkg.	68.9
APPLE BROWN BETTY	1 cup	63.9
APPLE BUTTER, cider		
(Smucker's)	1 T.	10.3
APPLE CIDER:		
Canned (Mott's) sweet	½ cup	14.6
*Mix, Country Time	8 fl. oz.	24.5
APPLE-CRANBERRY JUICE,		
Canned (Lincoln)	6 fl. oz.	26.0
APPLE DRINK:		
(Ann Page)	6 fl. oz.	20.0
(Hi-C)	6 fl. oz.	23.0
APPLE FRITTER (Mrs. Paul's)	2-oz. fritter	16.1
APPLE JACKS (Kellogg's)	1 cup	26.0
APPLE JELLY:		
Sweetened (Smucker's)	1 T.	13.3
Dietetic:		
(Dia-Mel) old-fashioned	1 T.	0
(Diet Delight)	1 T.	2.5
(Featherweight)	1 T.	3.0
APPLE JUICE:		
(Ann Page)	½ cup	20.0
(Lincoln)	6 fl. oz.	22.3
(Mott's) McIntosh	½ cup	14.6
APPLE PIE (See PIE, Apple)		
APPLE SAUCE:		
(Del Monte)	½ cup	23.6
(Mott's) natural	½ cup	26.2
Dietetic (Diet Delight)	½ cup	13.0
Dietetic (Featherweight)	½ cup	12.0
APPLE TURNOVER		
(Pillsbury)	1 turnover	26.0

Food and Description	Measure or Quantity	Carbohydrates (grams)
APRICOT:		
Fresh, whole	1 apricot	4.5
Canned:		
(Del Monte) whole, peeled	1 cup	50.0
(Libby's) heavy syrup, halves	1 cup	53.6
(Stokely-Van Camp)	1 cup	54.0
Dietetic:		
(Diet Delight) syrup pack	½ cup	15.0
(Diet Delight) water pack	½ cup	9.0
(Featherweight) juice pack	½ cup	12.0
Dried (Del Monte)	½ cup	39.9
APRICOT LIQUEUR (De Kuyper)	1 fl. oz.	8.3
APRICOT PRESERVE:		
Sweetened (Bama, Smucker's)	1 T.	12.7
Dietetic (Featherweight)	1 T.	4.0
APRICOT & PINEAPPLE PRESERVE:		
Sweetened (Smucker's)	1 T.	13.5
Dietetic (Diet Delight)	1 T.	2.3
APRICOT SOUR COCKTAIL (National Distillers-*Duet*)		
12½% alcohol	2 fl. oz.	1.6
AQUAVIT (Leroux)	1 fl. oz.	Tr.
ARTICHOKE:		
Boiled	12-oz. artichoke	42.1
Frozen (Birds Eye) hearts	3 oz.	5.5
Marinated, drained (Cara Mia)	6-oz. jar	7.2
ASPARAGUS:		
Boiled	1 spear (½″ dia. at base)	.7
Canned, spears, solids and liquid:		
(Del Monte) green	1 cup	6.4
(Del Monte) white	1 cup	7.3
(Green Giant) green	½ of 10½-oz. can	2.5
(Kounty Kist) green	½ of 15-oz. can	3.6
(Stokely-Van Camp)	1 cup	6.0
Dietetic (Diet Delight)	½ cup	2.3
Dietetic (Tillie Lewis)	½ cup	3.7
Frozen:		
(Birds Eye) cuts	⅓ pkg.	3.0
(Green Giant) cuts, butter sauce	1 cup	7.0
ASPARAGUS PUREE, dietetic (Cellu)	½ cup	3.5
*****ASPARAGUS SOUP** (Campbell)	10¾-oz. can	25.8
ASTI WINE (Gancia)	3 fl. oz.	18.0
AUNT JEMIMA SYRUP	¼ cup	54.0
AVOCADO, all varieties	1 fruit	14.3
*****AWAKE** (Birds Eye)	6 fl. oz.	21.2
AYDS, all flavors	1 piece	5.0

B

Food and Description	Measure or Quantity	Carbohydrates (grams)
BAC ONION (Lawry's)	1 tsp.	2.1
BACON, broiled:		
(Oscar Mayer) regular slice	7-gram slice	.1
(Oscar Mayer) thick slice	1 slice	.2
BACON BITS, imitation (Ann Page; Durkee; French's; McCormick)	1 tsp.	.5
BACON, CANADIAN, unheated (Oscar Mayer)	1-oz. slice	.2
BACON, SIMULATED, cooked, Sizzlean	1 strip	0
BAC*OS (General Mills)	1 T.	2.0
BAGEL (Lender's) garlic, onion or poppyseed	2-oz. bagel	31.5
BAKING POWDER (Calumet)	1 tsp.	1.0
BAMBOO SHOOTS:		
Raw, trimmed	¼ lb.	5.9
Canned (Chun King; La Choy) drained	½ of 8½-oz. can	3.6
BANANA, unpeeled, medium	6.2 oz. banana	26.4
BANANA ICE CREAM, red raspberry or strawberry twirl (Breyer's)	¼ pt.	21.0
BANANA PIE (See PIE, Banana)		
BARBECUE SEASONING (French's)	1 tsp.	1.0
BARDOLINO WINE (Antinori)	1 fl. oz.	6.3
BARLEY, pearled	¼ cup	39.4
BASIL (French's)	1 tsp.	.7
BASS:		
Baked, stuffed	3½″ x 4½″ x 1½″	23.4
Oven-fried	8¾″ x 4½″ x ⅝″	13.4
BAY LEAF (French's)	1 tsp.	1.0
B & B LIQUEUR	1 fl. oz.	5.7
B.B.Q. SAUCE & BEEF, frozen (Banquet) sliced beef, bag	5-oz. bag	12.5
BEAN, BAKED:		
(USDA) with pork & molasses sauce	1 cup	53.8
(USDA) with pork & tomato sauce	1 cup	48.5
(USDA) with tomato sauce	1 cup	58.7
(Ann Page) with pork & molasses sauce, Boston style	½ of 16-oz. can	49.8
(Ann Page) with pork & tomato sauce	½ of 16-oz. can	41.6
(Ann Page) vegetarian in tomato sauce	½ of 16-oz. can	44.1
(B&M) pea bean with pork in brown sugar sauce	8-oz. can	51.2
(B&M) red kidney bean in brown sugar sauce	½ of 16-oz. can	49.6

Food and Description	Measure or Quantity	Carbohydrates (grams)
(B&M) yellow eye bean in brown sugar sauce	½ of 16-oz. can	50.5
(Campbell) with pork, home style	½ of 16-oz. can	52.0
(Campbell) with molasses & brown sugar sauce, old fashioned	½ of 16-oz. can	49.0
(Campbell) with pork & tomato sauce	8-oz. can	44.0
(Homemaker's) red kidney in brown sugar sauce	1 cup	50.2
(Libby's) *deep brown* with pork & molasses sauce	½ of 14-oz. can	40.6
(Libby's) *deep brown* vegetarian in tomato sauce	½ of 14-oz. can	40.8
(Morton House) with tomato sauce	¼ of 16-oz. can	22.5
(Sultana) with pork & tomato sauce	½ of 16-oz. can	41.8
(Van Camp) with brown sugar sauce	1 cup	61.0
(Van Camp) with pork	1 cup	47.0
(Van Camp) vegetarian style	1 cup	48.0
BEAN & BEEF PATTIES (Swanson)	11-oz. dinner	16.0
BEAN & FRANKFURTER, canned (Campbell) in tomato and molasses sauce	8-oz. can	16.0
BEAN & FRANKFURTER DINNER:		
(Banquet)	10¾-oz. dinner	63.1
(Morton)	10¾-oz. dinner	79.4
(Swanson)	11¼-oz. dinner	75.0
BEAN, GREEN:		
Boiled, 1½" to 2" pieces, drained	½ cup	3.7
(Comstock) cut, drained	½ cup	2.4
(Del Monte) French, drained solids	½ cup	4.9
(Green Giant; Kounty Kist) French or whole, solids & liq.	½ cup	2.6
(Libby's) cut, solids & liq.	½ cup	4.1
(Libby's) French, solids & liq.	½ cup	4.2
(Stokely-Van Camp) solids & liq.	½ cup	3.5
Dietetic (Diet Delight) solids & liq.	½ cup	3.4
Frozen:		
(Birds Eye) cut	⅓ pkg.	5.0
(Birds Eye) with mushroom or onion	⅓ pkg.	6.0
(Birds Eye) with toasted almonds	⅓ pkg.	7.8
(Green Giant) in butter sauce	⅓ pkg.	3.0
(Green Giant) in mushroom sauce	⅓ pkg.	6.1

4

Food and Description	Measure or Quantity	Carbohydrates (grams)
BEAN, GREEN, PUREE, dietetic		
(Cellu)	½ cup	7.5
BEAN, ITALIAN:		
Canned (Del Monte) drained	½ cup	8.2
BEAN, KIDNEY:		
(Ann Page)	¼ of 15½-oz. can	19.3
(Ann Page) in chili gravy	½ of 15-oz. can	33.7
(Van Camp) red	1 cup	38.0
BEAN, LIMA:		
Boiled, drained	½ cup	16.8
(Del Monte) drained	½ cup	19.7
(Libby's) solids & liq.	½ cup	16.0
(Sultana) baby	¼ of 15-oz. can	12.0
(Sultana) butter bean	¼ of 15-oz. can	14.6
Dietetic (Featherweight) canned,		
solids & liq.	½ cup	16.0
Frozen:		
(Birds Eye) baby butter	⅓ pkg.	26.0
(Birds Eye) baby limas	⅓ pkg.	22.0
(Birds Eye) Fordhooks	⅓ pkg.	18.0
(Green Giant) baby limas	¼ pkg.	22.4
(Green Giant) speckled butter		
beans, Southern recipe	⅓ pkg.	13.2
(Kounty Kist) baby limas	⅕ pkg.	27.5
BEAN, RED MEXICAN (Green		
Giant)	¼ of 15½-oz. can	17.5
BEAN, REFRIED, canned		
(Ortega)	½ cup	25.0
BEAN SALAD (Green Giant)	4¼ oz.	19.9
BEAN SOUP:		
*(Ann Page) condensed, with		
bacon	1 cup	19.0
(Campbell) *Chunky,* with ham	11-oz. can	35.0
*(Campbell) condensed, with		
bacon	10-oz. serving	12.0
BEAN SOUP, BLACK:		
*(Campbell) condensed	8-oz. serving	24.2
(Crosse & Blackwell) with sherry	13-oz. can	36.0
BEAN SPROUT:		
Mung, raw	½ lb.	15.0
Mung, boiled, drained	¼ lb.	5.9
Soy, raw	½ lb.	12.0
Soy, boiled, drained	¼ lb.	4.2
Canned (Chun King) drained	½ of 16-oz. can	5.9
Canned (La Choy) drained	1 cup	1.3
BEAN, WHITE		
Great Northern, cooked	½ cup	18.0
BEAN, YELLOW OR WAX:		
Boiled, 1″ pieces, drained	½ cup	5.2
Canned:		
(Del Monte) cut, solids & liq.	½ cup	3.4
(Libby's) cut, solids & liq.	½ of 8-oz. can	4.4

Food and Description	Measure or Quantity	Carbohydrates (grams)
(Stokely-Van Camp) solids & liq.	½ cup	4.0
Dietetic (Featherweight) cut	½ cup	5.0
Frozen (Birds Eye) cut	⅓ pkg.	4.0
BEEF	Any quantity	0
BEEFAMATO COCKTAIL (Mott's)	½ cup	10.7
BEEF BOUILLON, MBT	1 packet	2.0
BEEF, CHIPPED:		
Cooked, home recipe	½ cup	8.7
Frozen, creamed (Banquet)	5-oz. pkg.	10.5
BEEF DINNER:		
(Banquet)	11-oz. dinner	20.9
(Morton)	10-oz. dinner	20.0
(Morton) Country Table, sliced	14-oz. dinner	63.7
(Morton) Steak House, tenderloin	9½-oz. dinner	45.9
(Morton) Steak House, sirloin strip	9½-oz. dinner	48.9
(Swanson) Hungry Man, chopped	18-oz. dinner	70.0
(Swanson) 3-course	15-oz. dinner	58.0
(Weight Watchers) beefsteak with pepper & mushrooms	10-oz. meal	11.1
(Weight Watchers) sirloin, 3-compartment	16-oz. meal	10.0
BEEF ENTREE, frozen		
(Swanson) Hungry Man, sliced	12¼-oz. entree	23.0
BEEF GOULASH (Bounty)	7½-oz. can	16.3
BEEF HASH, ROAST, canned		
(Hormel) Mary Kitchen	7½-oz.	9.0
BEEF JERKY (Lawry's)	¼-oz. piece	.1
BEEF PIE:		
(Banquet)	8-oz. pie	40.9
(Morton)	8-oz. pie	31.8
(Swanson)	8-oz. pie	43.0
(Swanson) Hungry Man	16-oz. pie	65.0
(Swanson) sirloin burger Hungry Man	16-oz. pie	55.0
BEEF PUFFS (Durkee)	1 piece	3.0
BEEF SOUP:		
*(Campbell) condensed	10-oz. serving	14.0
(Campbell) Chunky	10¾-oz. can	22.0
(Campbell) Chunky, low sodium	7½-oz. can	16.0
*(Campbell) consomme	10-oz. serving	4.0
*(Campbell) noodle	10-oz. serving	10.0
Dietetic (Dia-Mel) & noodle	8-oz. serving	5.0
Broth:		
*(Campbell) condensed	10-oz. serving	3.0
(College Inn)	1 cup	5.2
(Swanson)	½ of 13¾-oz. can	1.0
BEEF SOUP MIX:		
*(Lipton) Cup-a-Soup, noodle	6 fl. oz.	6.0
*(Nestlé's) Souptime	6 fl. oz.	4.0
*(Wyler's) noodle	6 fl. oz.	7.0

Food and Description	Measure or Quantity	Carbohydrates (grams)
BEEF STEW:		
Home recipe, made with lean beef chuck	1 cup	15.2
(Hormel) Dinty Moore	7½-oz. can	12.9
(Libby's)	1 cup	33.8
(Morton House)	½ of 24-oz. can	17.0
(Swanson)	½ of 15-oz. can	18.2
Dietetic (Dia-Mel)	8-oz. can	19.0
Dietetic (Featherweight)	7¼-oz. can	24.0
Frozen (Green Giant) & biscuits, Bake 'n Serve	14-oz. pkg.	40.6
BEEF STEW SEASONING MIX:		
(Durkee)	1 pkg.	22.0
(French's)	1 pkg.	36.0
BEEF STIX (Vienna)	1 oz.	1.4
BEEF STROGANOFF (Hormel)	½ of 1-lb. can	4.7
BEER & ALE:		
Regular, alcohol by volume:		
Black Horse Ale, 5% alcohol	8 fl. oz.	9.2
Black Label, 4.9 % alcohol	8 fl. oz.	7.5
Budweiser	8 fl. oz.	8.9
Busch Bavarian	8 fl. oz.	8.0
Heidelberg, 4.6% alcohol	8 fl. oz.	7.1
Knickerbocker, 4.6% alcohol	8 fl. oz.	9.1
Meister Brau Premium, regular or draft, 4.6% alcohol	8 fl. oz.	7.3
Michelob, 4.9% alcohol	8 fl. oz.	11.0
North Star, regular	8 fl. oz.	9.9
Old Milwaukee, 4.5% alcohol	8 fl. oz.	9.1
Pearl Premium, 4.7% alcohol	8 fl. oz.	8.3
Pfeifer, regular	8 fl. oz.	9.9
Pfeifer, 3.2 low gravity	8 fl. oz.	9.1
Red Cap, 5.6% alcohol	8 fl. oz.	7.2
Rheingold, 4.6% alcohol	8 fl. oz.	9.1
Schlitz, 4.9% alcohol	8 fl. oz.	9.1
Schlitz, repeal, 3.9% alcohol	8 fl. oz.	7.2
Schmidt, regular or extra special	8 fl. oz.	9.9
Schmidt, 3.2 low gravity	8 fl. oz.	9.1
Stag, 4.8% alcohol	8 fl. oz.	7.5
Tuborg, USA, 4.8% alcohol	8 fl. oz.	8.1
Light or low carbohydrate:		
Dia-beer	8 fl. oz.	2.8
Gablinger's, 4.5% alcohol	8 fl. oz.	.1
Meister Brau Lite, 4.6% alcohol	8 fl. oz.	.9
Michelob, light	8 fl. oz.	8.0
Natural Light	8 fl. oz.	4.0
Pearl Light, 2.9% alcohol	8 fl. oz.	1.0
Schlitz Light, 3.8% alcohol	8 fl. oz.	3.4
BEER, NEAR:		
Goetz Pale, 0.2% alcohol	8 fl. oz.	2.6
Kingsbury (Heilemann) 0.4% alcohol	8 fl. oz.	7.1

Food and Description	Measure or Quantity	Carbohydrates (grams)
(Metbrew) 0.4% alcohol	8 fl. oz.	9.1
BEET:		
Boiled, whole	2″ dia. beet	3.6
Boiled, sliced	½ cup	7.3
(Del Monte) pickled, solids & liq.	½ cup	18.1
(Del Monte) sliced, solids & liq.	½ cup	7.0
(Libby's) Harvard, solids & liq.	½ cup	20.8
(Stokely-Van Camp) pickled, solids & liq.	½ cup	22.5
Dietetic (Featherweight) sliced	½ cup	10.0
BEET PUREE, dietetic (Cellu)	½ cup	10.0
BENEDICTINE LIQUEUR (Julius Wile)	1½ fl. oz.	15.5
BIG H, burger sauce (Hellmann's)	1 T.	1.6
BIG MAC (See McDONALD'S)		
BIG WHEEL (Hostess)	1 cake	21.5
BISCUIT, egg (Stella D'oro)	1 biscuit	6.6
BISCUIT DOUGH:		
Baking powder (Pillsbury)		
1869 Brand Heat 'n Serve	1 piece	12.0
Buttermilk (Pillsbury)	1 piece	10.5
BI-SICLE (Popsicle Industries)	2½ fl. oz.	21.4
BITTERS (Angostura)	1 tsp.	2.0
BLACKBERRY, fresh, hulled	1 cup	18.8
BLACKBERRY BRANDY (DeKuyper)	1½ fl. oz.	10.3
BLACKBERRY JELLY:		
Sweetened (Smucker's)	1 T.	13.5
Dietetic (Featherweight)	1 T.	4.0
BLACKBERRY LIQUEUR (Bols)	1 fl. oz.	12.8
BLACKBERRY PRESERVE:		
Sweetened (Bama; Smucker's)	1 T.	13.7
Dietetic (Dia-Mel)	1 T.	0
Dietetic (Diet Delight; Featherweight)	1 T.	3.5
BLACKBERRY WINE (Mogen David)	3 fl. oz.	18.7
BLACK-EYED PEAS:		
Canned (Sultana) with pork	½ of 15-oz. can	33.9
Frozen:		
(Birds Eye)	⅓ pkg.	23.0
(Green Giant)	⅓ pkg.	12.7
BLACK RUSSIAN COCKTAIL MIX (Holland House)	1½ fl. oz.	34.5
BLOODY MARY MIX:		
Dry (Bar-Tender's)	1 serving	5.7
Liquid (Sacramento)	5½-fl.-oz. can	9.1
BLUEBERRY:		
Fresh	½ cup	11.2
Canned, dietetic (Featherweight) solids & liq.	½ cup	10.7

8

Food and Description	Measure or Quantity	Carbohydrates (grams)
BLUEBERRY PIE (See **PIE**, Blueberry)		
BLUEBERRY PRESERVE:		
Sweetened (Bama; Smucker's)	1 T.	13.7
Dietetic (Featherweight)	1 T.	4.0
BLUEBERRY TURNOVER (Pepperidge Farm)	1 turnover	32.0
BLUEFISH, broiled	1½″ x 3″ x ½″ piece	0
BOLOGNA:		
(Armour Star) all meat	1-oz. slice	0
(Hormel) all meat	1-oz. slice	.5
(Oscar Mayer) beef	.8-oz. slice	.7
(Oscar Mayer) Beef Lebanon	.8-oz. slice	.4
(Oscar Mayer) garlic beef	.8-oz. slice	.4
(Swift)	1-oz. slice	1.5
(Vienna) beef	1 oz.	.7
(Wilson)	1-oz. slice	.5
BORSCHT (Manischewitz)	½ cup	8.7
BOSCO, chocolate syrup	1 T.	13.3
BOYSENBERRY JELLY (Smucker's)	1 T.	13.7
BRAN, crude	1 oz.	17.5
BRAN BREAKFAST CEREAL:		
(Kellogg's):		
All-Bran	⅓ cup	22.0
Bran Buds	⅓ cup	23.0
Cracklin' Bran	⅓ cup	19.0
40% bran flakes	⅔ cup	23.0
Raisin	¾ cup	29.0
(Nabisco) 100% bran	½ cup	21.0
(Post) 40% bran flakes	⅔ cup	22.6
(Post) raisin	½ cup	22.0
(Ralston Purina) *Bran Chex*	⅔ cup	20.0
(Ralston Purina) raisin	½ cup	22.0
BRANDY, FLAVORED:		
Blackberry (Garnier; Hiram Walker)	1 fl. oz.	7.1
Cherry (Bols)	1 fl. oz.	7.4
BRAUNSCHWEIGER:		
(Oscar Mayer) tube	1 oz.	.7
(Swift) 8-oz. chub	1 oz.	1.4
(Wilson)	1 oz.	.7
BRAZIL NUT, shelled	4 nuts	1.9
BREAD:		
American Granary (Arnold)	.9-oz. slice	12.5
Boston Brown	3″ x ¾″ slice	21.9
Cracked wheat (Wonder)	1-oz. slice	13.5
Date-nut (Thomas')	1.1-oz. slice	18.4
Flatbread, *Ideal:*		
Ultra thin	.1-oz. slice	2.5
Whole grain	.2-oz. slice	4.0
French (Wonder)	1-oz. slice	13.5
Glutogen Gluten (Thomas')	.4-oz. slice	5.9
Hillbilly (Wonder)	1-oz. slice	12.5

Food and Description	Measure or Quantity	Carbohydrates (grams)
Hollywood	1-oz. slice	12.5
Honey, wheat berry (Arnold)	1.2-oz. slice	16.0
Italian (Pepperidge Farm)	2-oz. slice	28.0
Naturel (Arnold)	.9-oz. slice	12.0
Profile (Wonder) dark	.8-oz. slice	12.5
Protogen Protein (Thomas')	.7-oz. slice	8.3
Protogen Protein (Thomas') frozen	.9-oz. slice	10.2
Pumpernickle:		
(Arnold)	1-oz. slice	14.0
(Levy's)	1.1-oz. slice	12.4
(Pepperidge Farm)	1 slice	14.0
Raisin, cinnamon (Thomas')	.8-oz. slice	11.7
Raisin, orange (Arnold)	.9-oz. slice	12.6
Raisin, tea (Arnold)	.9-oz. slice	13.0
Roman Meal	1-oz. slice	13.5
Rye:		
(Arnold) Jewish	1.1-oz. slice	14.0
(Arnold) Jewish, *Dietslice*	.7-oz. slice	9.5
(Arnold) soft	1.1-oz. slice	15.0
(Pepperidge Farm) family	1 slice	14.5
Wasa:		
Golden	.4-oz. slice	7.8
Hearty	.5-oz. slice	11.4
Lite	.3-oz. slice	6.3
Seasoned	.3-oz. slice	7.1
(Wonder)	1-oz. slice	13.5
Sesame, *Wasa*	.5-oz. slice	9.0
Sour Dough, *Di Carlo*	1-oz. slice	13.5
Sourdough Toast, *Wasa*	.4-oz. slice	9.5
Sport, *Wasa*	.4-oz. slice	9.1
Wheat:		
Fresh Horizons	1-oz. slice	9.5
Home Pride	1-oz. slice	13.0
(Pepperidge Farm)	1 slice	17.0
Proclaim	1-oz. slice	11.0
(Wonder)	1-oz. slice	12.5
Wheatberry, *Home Pride*	1-oz. slice	12.5
White:		
(Arnold) *Brick Oven*	.8-oz. slice	11.0
(Arnold) Melba thin	.5-oz. slice	7.0
(Pepperidge Farm) sliced	.8-oz. slice	13.0
(Wonder) *Home Pride*	1-oz. slice	13.0
Whole wheat:		
(Arnold) *Brick Oven*	.8-oz. slice	9.5
(Arnold) Melba thin	.5-oz. slice	6.5
(Pepperidge Farm) thin slice	.9-oz. slice	12.0
(Thomas'), 100%	.8-oz. slice	10.1
BREAD, CANNED, brown, plain or raisin (B&M)	1-oz. slice	11.4
BREAD CRUMBS (Contadina) seasoned	½ cup	44.3

Food and Description	Measure or Quantity	Carbohydrates (grams)
*BREAD DOUGH (Rich's):		
French	1/20 of loaf	11.0
Italian	1/20 of loaf	11.0
Raisin	1/20 of loaf	12.3
*BREAD MIX (Pillsbury):		
Apricot, nut, banana or blueberry nut	1/16 of loaf	20.0
Cranberry and date	1/16 of loaf	22.0
BREAD PUDDING, with raisins	1/2 cup	37.6
BREAD STICK:		
Cheese, onion or salt (Keebler)	2 pieces	3.6
Dietetic or regular (Stella D'oro)	1 piece	6.3
BREAKFAST BAR (Carnation) all flavors	1 piece	20.0
BREAKFAST DRINK:		
(Ann Page)	2 tsps.	15.9
*(Pillsbury)	1 pouch	26.0
BREAKFAST SQUARES (General Mills) all flavors)	2 bars	45.0
BRIGHT & EARLY	6 fl. oz.	21.6
BROCCOLI:		
Boiled, whole stalk	1 stalk	8.1
Boiled, 1/2" pieces	1/2 cup	3.5
Frozen:		
(Birds Eye) in cheese sauce	1/3 pkg.	8.0
(Birds Eye) in Hollandaise sauce	1/3 pkg.	2.9
(Green Giant) spears in butter sauce	1/3 pkg.	3.7
(Green Giant) in cheese sauce, Bake 'n Serve	1/3 pkg.	5.6
(Green Giant) in cream sauce	1/2 cup	8.5
(Mrs. Paul's) in cheese sauce	1/3 pkg.	18.6
BROTH & SEASONING:		
(George Washington)	1 packet	1.0
Maggi	1 T.	.1
BRUSSELS SPROUT:		
Boiled	3-4 sprouts	4.9
Frozen:		
(Birds Eye)	1/3 pkg.	5.0
(Birds Eye) baby sprouts	1/3 pkg.	5.8
(Green Giant) butter sauce	1/3 pkg.	5.0
(Green Giant) halves in cheese sauce	1/3 pkg.	6.6
(Kounty Kist)	1/5 pkg.	7.3
BUCKWHEAT, cracked (Pocono)	1 oz.	19.4
BUC*WHEATS, cereal (General Mills)	1 oz.	23.0
BULGUR, canned, seasoned	4 oz.	37.2
BURGER KING:		
Cheeseburger	1 burger	26.0
Cheeseburger, double meat	1 burger	26.0

Food and Description	Measure or Quantity	Carbohydrates (grams)
French fries	1 small order	28.0
Hamburger	1 burger	25.0
Hamburger, double meat	1 burger	25.0
Hot dog	1 piece	24.0
Onion rings	1 small order	20.0
Whaler	1 sandwich	66.0
Whaler, with cheese	1 sandwich	66.0
Whopper:		
Plain	1 burger	50.0
Cheese	1 burger	51.0
Double meat	1 burger	50.0
Double meat with cheese	1 burger	51.0
Junior	1 burger	26.0
Junior with cheese	1 burger	26.0
Junior double meat	1 burger	26.0
Junior double meat with cheese	1 burger	26.0
Yumbo	1 sandwich	31.0
BURGUNDY WINE:		
(Gallo) regular or hearty	3 fl. oz.	1.2
(Great Western)	3 fl. oz.	2.3
(Inglenook) Navalle	3 fl. oz.	1.7
(Italian Swiss Colony)	3 fl. oz.	.9
(Louis M. Martini)	3 fl. oz.	.2
(Petri)	3 fl. oz.	1.3
(Taylor)	3 fl. oz.	3.3
BURGUNDY WINE, SPARKLING:		
(B&G)	3 fl. oz.	2.2
(Great Western)	3 fl. oz.	5.1
(Taylor)	3 fl. oz.	4.2
BUTTER:		
Regular (Breakstone)	1 T.	<.1
Regular (Meadow Gold)	1 tsp.	0
Whipped (Breakstone)	1 T.	.1
BUTTERNUT, shelled	1 oz.	2.4
BUTTER PECAN ICE CREAM		
(Breyer's)	¼ pt.	15.0
BUTTERSCOTCH MORSELS		
(Nestlé)	1 oz.	19.0

C

CABBAGE:		
Red, sweet & sour (Greenwood's)	½ cup	13.6
White, chopped	½ cup	4.4
Frozen (Green Giant) stuffed	7 oz.	16.5
CAFE COMFORT, 55 proof	1 fl. oz.	8.8
CAKE:		
Plain:		
Home recipe, with butter, without icing	⅑ of 9″ sq. cake	48.1

Food and Description	*Measure or Quantity*	*Carbohydrates (grams)*
Home recipe, with butter, with chocolate icing	1/9 of 9″ square	73.1
Angel Food, home recipe	1/12 of 8″ cake	24.1
Banana, frozen (Sara Lee)	1/8 of cake	26.8
Banana, frozen (Sara Lee) *Light 'n Luscious*	1/8 of cake	19.1
Banana nut, frozen (Sara Lee) layer	1/8 of cake	26.5
Caramel:		
Home recipe, without icing	1/9 of 9″ square	46.2
Home recipe, with caramel icing	1/9 of 9″ square	50.2
Cheesecake, frozen:		
(Rich's)	1/16 of cake	19.6
(Sara Lee):		
Cherry cream cheese	1/6 of cake	30.3
Cream cheese, small	1/3 of cake	28.3
Strawberry cream cheese	1/6 of cake	30.0
Chocolate:		
Home recipe, with chocolate icing, 2-layer	1/12 of 9″ cake	55.2
Frozen:		
(Pepperidge Farm) fudge	1/6 of cake	43.4
(Sara Lee)	1/8 of cake	24.3
(Sara Lee) *Light 'n Luscious*	1/8 of cake	19.6
(Sara Lee) 'n cream, layer	1/8 of cake	23.8
(Sara Lee) double chocolate, layer	1/8 of cake	24.0
(Sara Lee) German	1/8 of cake	17.3
Coffee:		
(Drake's):		
Junior	1 cake (1.1 oz.)	18.4
Pecan ring	13-oz. ring	210.8
Raspberry ring	13-oz. ring	199.6
Small	1 cake (2.4 oz.)	40.3
Frozen:		
(Pepperidge Farm) cinnamon twist	1/6 of cake (1.8 oz.)	21.3
(Sara Lee):		
Almond	1/8 of cake	19.3
Apple Fruit 'n Danish	1/8 of cake	18.8
Blueberry ring	1/8 of cake	17.6
Cinnamon	1/8 of cake	18.1
Maple crunch ring	1/8 of cake	15.6
Pecan, large	1/8 of cake	18.0
Streusel, large	1/8 of cake	16.6
Crumb, frozen (Sara Lee):		
Blueberry	1 cake	23.9
French	1 cake	27.0
Devil's Food, frozen:		
Home recipe, without icing	3″ x 2″ x 1½″ piece	28.6
Frozen:		
(Pepperidge Farm)	1/6 of cake	47.0

Food and Description	Measure or Quantity	Carbohydrates (grams)
(Sara Lee)	⅛ of cake	25.1
Fruit:		
Home recipe, dark	⅟₃₀ of 8″ loaf	9.0
Home recipe, light, made with butter	⅟₃₀ of 8″ loaf	8.6
Orange, frozen (Sara Lee)	⅛ of cake	25.3
Pound:		
Home recipe, equal weights flour, sugar, butter & eggs	3½″ x 3½″ slice (1.1 oz.)	14.1
Home recipe, traditional, made with butter	3½″ x 3½″ slice (1.1 oz.)	16.4
(Drake's):		
Plain	1 slice (1.6 oz.)	25.1
All butter, junior	1 slice (1.2 oz.)	19.2
Frozen (Sara Lee):		
Regular	⅟₁₀ of cake	14.4
Chocolate	⅟₁₀ of cake	13.0
Chocolate swirl	⅟₁₀ of cake	17.9
Home style	⅟₁₀ of cake	12.7
Sponge, home recipe	⅟₁₂ of 10″ cake	35.7
Strawberry shortcake, frozen (Sara Lee)	⅛ of cake	25.9
White:		
Home recipe, made with butter, without icing, 2-layer	⅑ of 9″ wide, 3″ high cake	50.8
Home recipe, made with butter, with coconut icing, 2-layer	⅟₁₂ of 9″ wide, 3″ high cake	63.1
Yellow:		
Home recipe, made with butter, with chocolate icing, 2-layer	⅟₁₂ of 9″ cake	60.4
(Sara Lee) frozen, *Light 'n Luscious*	⅛ of cake	21.7
CAKE ICING:		
Butter pecan (Betty Crocker) ready to spread	⅟₁₂ of can	27.0
Chocolate:		
Home recipe (USDA)	4 oz.	76.4
Ready to spread:		
(Betty Crocker)	⅟₁₂ of can	25.0
(Betty Crocker) nut	⅟₁₂ of can	24.0
(Pillsbury) milk	⅟₁₂ pkg.	24.0
Coconut, home recipe (USDA)	4 oz.	84.9
Double Dutch (Pillsbury) ready to spread	⅟₁₂ pkg.	24.0
Lemon (Pillsbury) ready to spread	⅟₁₂ pkg.	27.0
Orange (Betty Crocker) ready to spread	⅟₁₂ of can	26.0

Food and Description	Measure or Quantity	Carbohydrates (grams)
Sour cream chocolate (Betty Crocker) ready to spread	1/12 of can	25.0
Strawberry (Pillsbury) ready to spread	1/12 pkg.	27.0
Vanilla (Pillsbury), ready to spread	1/12 pkg.	27.0
White:		
Home recipe, boiled (USDA)	4 oz.	91.1
Home recipe, uncooked (USDA)	4 oz.	92.5
*CAKE ICING MIX:		
Banana (Betty Crocker) *Chiquita*, creamy	1/12 of cake's icing	30.0
Butter pecan (Betty Crocker) creamy	1/12 of cake's icing	30.0
Caramel (Pillsbury) *Rich 'n Easy*	1/12 of cake's icing	29.0
Chocolate chip (Betty Crocker) creamy	1/12 of cake's icing	32.0
Chocolate:		
Fudge:		
Home recipe (USDA)	4 oz.	76.0
(Betty Crocker) creamy	1/12 of cake's icing	32.0
(Pillsbury) *Rich 'n Easy*	1/12 of cake's icing	30.0
Milk (Pillsbury) *Rich 'n Easy*	1/12 of cake's icing	29.0
Whipped (Betty Crocker)	1/12 of cake's icing	18.0
Coconut pecan (Pillsbury)	1/12 of cake's icing	20.0
Double Dutch (Pillsbury) *Nice 'n Easy*	1/12 of cake's icing	30.0
Fudge:		
Home recipe, prepared with water, creamy (USDA)	4 oz.	84.6
(Betty Crocker) dark chocolate	1/12 of cake's icing	30.0
Lemon:		
(Betty Crocker) *Sunkist*, creamy	1/12 of cake's icing	30.0
(Pillsbury) *Rich 'n Easy*	1/12 of cake's icing	30.0
Orange (Betty Crocker) creamy	1/12 of cake's icing	30.0
Spice (Betty Crocker) creamy	1/12 of cake's icing	30.0
Sour cream white (Betty Crocker) creamy	1/12 of cake's icing	30.0
Strawberry cream (Betty Crocker) whipped	1/12 of cake's icing	18.0
Vanilla (Betty Crocker) whipped	1/12 of cake's icing	18.0
White (Betty Crocker) creamy	1/12 of cake's icing	33.0
CAKE MIX:		
Angel Food:		
*(USDA)	1/12 of 10" cake	31.5
(Betty Crocker):		
Chocolate	1/12 pkg.	32.0
One-step	1/12 pkg.	32.0
Traditional	1/12 pkg.	30.0
(Duncan Hines)	1/12 pkg.	28.9
*(Pillsbury) white	1/12 of cake	33.0
*(Swans Down)	1/12 of cake	29.7

Food and Description	Measure or Quantity	Carbohydrates (grams)
Banana Nut (Duncan Hines)		
Moist & Easy Snack Cake	⅑ pkg.	31.0
Banana Walnut (Betty Crocker)		
Snackin' Cake	⅑ pkg.	33.0
*Butter Pecan (Betty Crocker) layer	¹⁄₁₂ of cake	34.0
Cheesecake:		
*(Betty Crocker) cherry fudge	¹⁄₁₂ of cake	34.0
*(Jell-O)	⅛ of 8″ cake	33.0
*(Pillsbury) no bake	⅛ of cake	34.0
*(Royal)	⅛ of cake	31.0
Chocolate:		
(Betty Crocker):		
Chip, *Snackin' Cake*	⅑ pkg.	35.0
Fudge, *Snackin' Cake*	⅑ pkg.	34.0
*German chocolate, layer	¹⁄₁₂ of cake	34.0
*Milk, layer	¹⁄₁₂ of cake	34.0
*Pudding	⅙ of cake	45.0
(Duncan Hines):		
Chip, *Moist & Easy Snack Cake*	⅑ pkg.	32.7
Chip, golden, *Moist & Easy Snack Cake*	⅑ pkg.	32.7
*(Pillsbury):		
Dark, *Pillsbury Plus*	¹⁄₁₂ of cake	33.0
German, *Pillsbury Plus*	¹⁄₁₂ of cake	33.0
*Cinnamon (Pillsbury), *Streusel Swirl*	¹⁄₁₂ of cake	51.0
Coffee cake:		
*(Aunt Jemima)	⅛ of cake	29.0
*(Pillsbury):		
Apple cinnamon	⅛ of cake	40.0
Cinnamon streusel	⅛ of cake	41.0
Sour Cream	⅛ of cake	35.0
Devil's Food:		
*(Betty Crocker) layer, butter recipe	¹⁄₁₂ of cake	35.0
(Duncan Hines) *Pudding Recipe*	¹⁄₁₂ pkg.	34.8
*(Pillsbury):		
Bundt Basic	¹⁄₁₂ of cake	34.0
Streusel Swirl	¹⁄₁₂ of cake	50.0
*Fudge:		
*(Pillsbury):		
Bundt ring, triple fudge	¹⁄₁₂ of cake	42.0
Streusel Swirl, marble	¹⁄₁₂ of cake	51.0
Lemon:		
*(Betty Crocker) pudding	⅙ of cake	45.0
(Duncan Hines) *Pudding Recipe*	¹⁄₁₂ pkg.	36.1
*(Pillsbury):		
Bundt Basic	¹⁄₁₂ of cake	35.0
Pillsbury Plus	¹⁄₁₂ of cake	33.0

Food and Description	Measure or Quantity	Carbohydrates (grams)
Marble:		
*(Betty Crocker) layer	1/12 of cake	36.0
*(Pillsbury) Supreme, *Bundt* ring	1/12 of cake	51.0
Pound:		
*(Betty Crocker) golden	1/12 of cake	27.0
*(Dromedary)	1" slice	46.0
Spice (Betty Crocker):		
*'N Apple with raisin, layer	1/12 of cake	37.0
*Sour cream, layer	1/12 of cake	34.0
*Upside down cake (Betty Crocker) pineapple	1/9 of cake	42.0
White:		
(Duncan Hines) *Pudding Recipe*	1/12 pkg.	36.5
*(Pillsbury) *Pillsbury Plus*	1/12 of cake	36.0
Yellow:		
*(Betty Crocker) layer	1/12 of cake	35.0
(Duncan Hines) *Pudding Recipe*	1/12 pkg.	37.0
*(Pillsbury) *Bundt Basic*	1/12 of cake	36.0
*(Pillsbury) *Pillsbury Plus* butter recipe	1/12 of cake	33.0
Dietetic (Dia-Mel) all flavors	1/10 of cake	18.0
CANDY, REGULAR:		
Almond, chocolate covered, *Golden Almond* (Hershey's)	1 oz.	12.4
Baby Ruth (Curtiss)	1.8-oz. piece	31.0
Baffle Bar (Cardinet's)	1¾-oz. bar	10.9
Breath Saver (Life Savers)	1 piece	1.7
Bridge Mix (Nabisco)	1 piece	1.4
Bun Bars (Wayne)	1 oz.	17.0
Butterfinger (Curtiss)	1.6-oz. bar	28.0
Butternut (Hollywood)	1¼-oz. bar	20.6
Butterscotch Skimmers (Nabisco)	1 piece	5.7
Candy corn (Brach's)	1 piece	1.8
Caramel:		
Caramel Flipper (Wayne)	1 oz.	19.0
Caramel Nip (Pearson)	1 piece	5.6
(Curtiss)	1 piece	5.0
Charleston Chew	1½-oz. bar	32.6
Cherry, chocolate-covered (Brach's; Nabisco)	1 piece	13.2
Chocolate bar:		
Choco-Lite (Nestlé)	.35-oz. miniature	6.3
Choco-Lite (Nestlé)	1-oz. bar	18.0
Milk:		
(Hershey's)	1.2-oz. bar	19.4
(Hershey's)	4-oz. bar	64.7
(Nestlé)	.35-oz. miniature	6.0
(Nestlé)	1⅛-oz. bar	27.6
Special Dark (Hershey's)	1.05-oz. bar	18.4
Special Dark (Hershey's)	4-oz. bar	70.2

Food and Description	Measure or Quantity	Carbohydrates (grams)
Chocolate bar with almonds:		
(Hershey's) milk	.35-oz. miniature	5.4
(Hershey's) milk	1.15-oz. bar	17.6
(Hershey's) milk	4-oz. bar	61.4
(Nestlé)	1-oz. serving	17.0
(Nestlé)	5-oz. bar	85.0
Chocolate Parfait (Pearson)	1 piece	5.2
Chuckles	1 oz.	23.0
Circus Peanuts (Curtiss)	1 piece	6.0
Coconut bar, *Welch's* (Nabisco)	1 piece	21.8
Coffee Nip (Pearson)	1 piece	5.6
Coffioca (Pearson)	1 piece	5.2
Crows (Mason)	1 piece	2.7
Dots (Mason)	1 piece	2.7
Fiddle Faddle	1½-oz. packet	34.7
Forever Yours (M&M/Mars)	1.4-oz. bar	28.6
Frappe (Welch's)	1 piece	23.5
Fruit Roll (Sahadi):		
Any flavor but strawberry	1 oz.	20.0
Strawberry	1 oz.	22.0
Fudge, nut, bars or squares (Nabisco)	1 piece	10.2
Good & Fruity	1 oz.	26.3
Good & Plenty	1 oz.	24.8
Hard candy (Pearson) Grape suckers	1 piece	21.0
Hollywood	1½-oz. bar	28.9
Jujubes (Nabisco)	1 piece	3.3
Ju Jus:		
Assorted	1 piece	2.0
Coins or raspberries	1 piece	4.0
Kisses (Hershey's)	1 piece	2.8
Kit Kat	.6-oz. miniature	9.4
Kit Kat	1⅛-oz. bar	21.0
Krackel Bar	.35-oz. miniature	5.9
Krackel Bar	1.2-oz. bar	20.3
Krackel Bar	4-oz. bar	67.7
Licorice:		
Licorice Nips (Pearson)	1 piece	5.6
Twist:		
Black (American Licorice Co.)	1 piece	6.4
Black (Curtiss)	1 piece	6.0
Red (American Licorice Co.)	1 piece	7.3
Life Savers, drop	1 piece	2.4
Life Savers, mint	1 piece	1.7
Lollipops (Life Savers)	.9-oz. pop	24.0
Lollipops (Life Savers)	.6-oz. pop	16.7
Malted Milk Balls (Brach's)	1 piece	1.6
Marathon (M&M/Mars, Snackmaster)	.4-oz. bar	8.5
Mars Almond Bar (M&M/Mars)	1¼-oz. bar	22.1
Marshmallow (Campfire)	1 piece	24.9

Food and Description	Measure or Quantity	Carbohydrates (grams)
Mary Jane (Miller):		
2¢ size	1 piece	3.3
15¢ size	1 piece	19.5
Milk Shake (Hollywood)	1¼-oz. bar	26.8
Milky Way (M&M/Mars)	.8-oz. fun bar	15.5
Milky Way (M&M/Mars)	1.8-oz. bar	35.1
Milky Way (M&M/Mars)	2¼-oz. bar	43.7
Mint or peppermint:		
After dinner (Richardson):		
Jelly center	1 oz.	26.0
Regular	1 oz.	27.0
Chocolate-covered (Richardson)	1 oz.	27.0
Cool Mints (Curtiss)	1 piece	5.0
Jamaica or Liberty Mints (Nabisco)	1 piece	5.8
Mighty Mint (Life Savers)	1 piece	.4
Mint Parfait (Pearson)	1 piece	5.2
Junior mint pattie (Nabisco)	1 piece	2.0
Peppermint pattie (Nabisco)	1 piece	12.5
Thin (Nabisco)	1 piece	8.1
M & M's:		
Peanut	1 oz.	16.3
Plain	1 oz.	19.3
Mr. Goodbar (Hershey's)	.35-oz. miniature	4.9
Mr. Goodbar (Hershey's)	1½-oz. bar	20.8
Mr. Goodbar (Hershey's)	4-oz. bar	55.6
Munch peanut bar (M&M/Mars, Snack-master)	1½-oz. bar	19.0
Nib Nax (Y&S) all flavors	1 piece	2.5
Nibs (Y & S) all flavors	1 piece	1.5
$100,000 Bar (Nestlé)	1⅛-oz. bar	21.4
Orange slices (Curtiss)	1 piece	14.4
Orange slices (Nabisco) Chuckles	1 piece	7.2
Payday (Hollywood)	1⅛-oz. bar	22.3
Peanut, chocolate-covered:		
(Brach's)	1 piece	1.0
(Curtiss)	1 piece	1.0
(Nabisco)	1 piece	1.6
Peanut, French burnt (Curtiss)	1 piece	1.0
Peanut brittle (Planters):		
Jumbo Peanut Block Bar	1 oz.	23.0
Jumbo Peanut Block Bar	1 piece (.4 grams)	12.0
Peanut butter cup:		
(Boyer)	1.5-oz. pkg.	17.4
(Reese's)	.6-oz. cup	8.7
Pom Poms (Nabisco)	1 piece	2.3
Raisin, chocolate-covered:		
(Curtiss)	1 oz.	20.0
(Nabisco)	1 piece	.6
Raisinets (BB)	5¢ size	15.4
Reggie Bar	2-oz. bar	29.0
Rolo (Hershey's)	1 piece	4.1

Food and Description	Measure or Quantity	Carbohydrates (grams)
Sesame Crunch (Sahadi)	¾-oz. bar	9.0
Snickers	.8-oz. bar	14.5
Snickers	1.8-oz. bar	32.9
Spearmint leaves:		
(Curtiss)	1 piece	8.0
(Nabisco) Chuckles	1 piece	6.6
Starburst (M&M/Mars)	1-oz. serving	26.7
Stars, chocolate (Nabisco)	1 piece	1.6
Sugar Babies (Nabisco)	1 piece	1.3
Sugar Daddy (Nabisco):		
Caramel sucker	1 piece	26.4
Nugget	1 piece	6.0
Sugar Mama (Nabisco)	1 piece	18.6
Sugar Wafer (F & F)	1¼-oz. pkg.	26.0
Summit, cookie bar (M&M/Mars)	1.4-oz. serving	21.9
Taffy:		
Salt water (Brach's)	1 piece	6.8
Turkish (Bonomo)	1-oz. bar	24.4
3 Muskateers	.8-oz. fun bar	17.4
3 Muskateers	2.1-oz. bar	44.7
Toffee (Kraft) all flavors	1 piece	5.2
Tootsie Roll:		
Chocolate	.23-oz. midgee	5.3
Chocolate	1/16-oz. bar	14.3
Chocolate	¾-oz. bar	17.2
Chocolate	1-oz. bar	22.9
Chocolate	1¾-oz. bar	40.0
Flavored	.6-oz. square	3.8
Pop, all flavors	.49-oz. pop	12.5
Pop drop, all flavors	4.7-gram piece	4.2
Twix, cookie bar (M&M/Mars)	1¾-oz. bar	31.3
Twizzlers (Y & S):		
Licorice	1 oz.	24.0
Strawberry bars	1¼ oz.	30.0
U-No Bar (Cardinet's)	⅞-oz. bar	9.3
World Series Bar	1 oz.	21.3
CANDY, DIETETIC:		
Assorted, Sug'r Like	1 piece	3.0
Chocolate bar with almonds (Estee)	¾-oz. bar	9.6
Chocolate bar, bittersweet (Estee)	1 section of 3-oz. bar	3.3
Chocolate bar, crunch (Estee)	1 section of 2½-oz. bar	2.9
Chocolate bar, fruit & nut (Estee)	1 section of 3-oz. bar	3.2
Chocolate bar, milk (Estee)	¾-oz. bar	10.2
Gum drops:		
(Estee)	1 piece	.8
Sug'r Like, all flavors	1 piece	1.0
Hard candy:		
(Estee)	1 piece	3.0
Slimtreats	1 piece	0
Sug'r Like, all flavors	1 piece	3.0
Mint:		
(Estee)	1 piece	1.0

Food and Description	Measure or Quantity	Carbohydrates (grams)
Sug'r Like	1 piece	DNA
Peanut butter cup (Estee)	1 cup	2.9
Raisins, chocolate-covered (Estee)	1 piece	.7
TV Mix (Estee)	1 piece	.7
CANTALOUPE, Cubed	½ cup	6.1
CAPERS (Crosse & Blackwell)	1 tsp.	.3
CAP'N CRUNCH, cereal, regular (Quaker)	¾ cup	22.9
CARAWAY SEED (French's)	1 tsp.	.8
CARNATION INSTANT BREAKFAST	1 pkg.	23.0
CARROT:		
Raw	5½" x 1" carrot	4.8
Boiled, slices	½ cup	5.4
Canned:		
(Del Monte) drained	½ cup	6.8
(Libby's) solids & liq.	½ cup	4.5
(Stokely-Van Camp) solids & liq.	½ cup	5.0
Dietetic (Featherweight) solids & liq.	½ cup	6.0
Frozen:		
(Birds Eye) with brown sugar glaze	⅓ pkg.	14.6
(Green Giant) nuggets in butter sauce	⅓ pkg.	6.0
CARROT JUICE, canned (Diamond A)	½ cup	7.1
CARROT PUREE, dietetic (Cellu)	½ cup	7.5
CASABA MELON	1-lb. melon	14.7
CASHEW NUT:		
(A&P) dry roasted	1 oz.	7.3
(Planters) dry roasted	1 oz.	9.0
(Planters) oil roasted	1 oz.	8.0
(Tom Houston)	15 nuts	8.8
CATSUP:		
(Del Monte)	1 T.	5.5
(Hunt's)	1 T.	5.8
Dietetic (Dia-Mel; Featherweight)	1 T.	1.2
CAULIFLOWER:		
Raw or boiled buds	½ cup	2.6
Frozen:		
(Birds Eye)	⅓ pkg.	3.7
(Green Giant) in cheese sauce, *Bake 'n Serve*	⅓ pkg.	5.6
(Mrs. Paul's) light batter & cheese	⅓ pkg.	15.4
CAVIAR:		
Pressed	1 oz.	1.4
Whole eggs	1 T.	.5
CELERY:		
1 large outer stalk	8" x 1½" at root end	1.6

21

Food and Description	Measure or Quantity	Carbohydrates (grams)
Diced or cut	½ cup	2.1
Seed (French's)	1 tsp.	1.1
*CELERY SOUP, cream of:		
(Ann Page)	1 cup	8.3
(Campbell)	1 cup	8.0
CERTS	1 piece	1.5
CHABLIS WINE:		
(B&G; Inglenook-Navalle)	3 fl. oz.	.1
(Gallo)	3 fl. oz.	3.0
(Great Western)	3 fl. oz.	2.3
CHAMPAGNE:		
(Bollinger)	3 fl. oz.	3.6
(Gold Seal) pink, extra dry	3 fl. oz.	2.6
(Great Western):		
Regular	3 fl. oz.	2.4
Brut	3 fl. oz.	3.4
Extra dry	3 fl. oz.	4.3
Pink	3 fl. oz.	4.9
(Lejon)	3 fl. oz.	2.5
(Mumm's) Cordon Rouge, brut	3 fl. oz.	1.4
(Mumm's) extra dry	3 fl. oz.	5.6
(Taylor) dry	3 fl. oz.	3.9
CHARLOTTE RUSSE, homemade recipe	4 oz.	38.0
*CHEDDAR CHEESE SOUP (Campbell)	8-oz. serving	9.6
CHEERIOS, cereal	1 oz.	20.0
CHEESE:		
American or cheddar:		
Natural:		
Cube	1″ cube	.4
(Kraft)	1 oz.	.6
(Sealtest) cheddar	1 oz.	.6
Wispride, sharp cheddar	1 T.	1.5
Process:		
(Borden)	¾-oz. slice	1.2
(Kraft)	1-oz. slice	.5
(Borden) *Miracle Melt*	1 T.	.6
American blue (Borden) *Miracle Melt*	1 T.	.5
Asiago (Frigo)	1 oz.	.6
Blue:		
(Frigo)	1 oz.	.5
(Kraft)	1 oz.	.5
Brick (Kraft) natural	1 oz.	.3
Camembert	1 oz.	.5
Caraway (Kraft) natural	1 oz.	.6
Colby:		
(Borden; Kraft)	1 oz.	.6
Low sodium (Cellu)	1 oz.	0
Low sodium (Pauly)	1 oz.	.6

Food and Description	Measure or Quantity	Carbohydrates (grams)
Cottage:		
Creamed, unflavored:		
(Axelrod; Dean)	8-oz. container	3.5
(Borden) *Lite Line*	1 cup	7.0
(Breakstone) California	8-oz. container	4.8
(Breakstone) tangy tiny curd	8-oz. container	4.8
(Frigo)	8-oz. serving	6.4
(Sealtest)	1 cup	8.0
(Sealtest) *Light 'n Lively*	1 cup	5.6
Creamed, flavored:		
Garden salad, *Light 'n Lively*	1 cup	10.0
Garden salad (Sealtest)	1 cup	10.0
Peach-pineapple, *Light 'n Lively*	1 cup	22.0
Peach-pineapple (Sealtest)	1 cup	17.9
Uncreamed:		
(Breakstone) pot	8-oz. container	3.9
(Breakstone) skim milk	8-oz. container	1.6
(Dean)	8-oz. container	3.6
(Frigo) part skim milk	8-oz. serving	6.4
Cream cheese:		
Plain, unwhipped:		
(Borden)	1 oz.	1.5
(Breakstone; Kraft-*Hostess;* Sealtest)	1 oz.	.6
(Kraft) *Philadelphia*	1 oz.	.9
(Kraft) *Philadelphia,* imitation	1 oz.	1.9
Plain, whipped (Breakstone) *Temp-Tee*	1 T.	.2
Flavored, unwhipped:		
Pimiento (Bordon)	1 oz.	.6
Chive or olive-pimiento (Kraft) *Hostess*	1 oz.	.8
Flavored, whipped (Kraft) *Philadelphia:*		
Bacon & horseradish	1 oz.	1.3
Onion, pimiento	1 oz.	1.9
Smoked salmon	1 oz.	1.1
Edam (House of Gold)	1 oz.	.3
Farmer (Dean)	1 oz.	.7
Farmer, *Wispride*	1 oz.	1.0
Gorgonzola (Foremost Blue Moon)	1 oz.	Tr.
Gouda:		
(Borden) Dutch Maid	1 oz.	.5
(Foremost Blue Moon) baby	1 oz.	Tr.
(Kraft) natural	1 oz.	.5
Gruyere:		
(Borden)	1 oz.	1.4
(Kraft)	1 oz.	.6
Swiss Knight	1 oz.	.5
Kisses (Borden)	1 piece	.5
Liederkranz (Borden)	1 oz.	.4

Food and Description	Measure or Quantity	Carbohydrates (grams)
Limburger (Borden-*Dutch Maid*; Kraft)	1 oz.	.6
Lite-Line (Bordon)	¾-oz. slice	.8
Monterey Jack (Frigo; Kraft)	1 oz.	.4
Mozzarella:		
(Borden)	1 oz.	.8
(Kraft)	1 oz.	.3
Muenster, natural:		
(Borden)	1 oz.	.7
(Kraft)	1 oz.	.3
Neufchâtel (Kraft) loaf	1 oz.	.7
Old English (Kraft)	1 oz.	.5
Parmesan:		
Grated:		
(Borden)	1 oz.	8.8
(Kraft)	1 oz.	1.0
Shredded (Kraft)	1 oz.	.9
& Romano, grated:		
(Borden) natural	1 oz.	2.2
(Kraft)	1 oz.	1.0
Pepato (Frigo)	1 oz.	.8
Pimiento American, process (Borden; Kraft)	1 oz.	.5
Pizza:		
(Borden)	1 oz.	.8
(Frigo)	1 oz.	.3
Port du Salut (Foremost Blue Moon)	1 oz.	Tr.
Provolone:		
(Borden)	1 oz.	1.0
(Frigo)	1 oz.	.5
Ricotta (Frigo) part skim milk	1 oz.	.9
Ricotta (Sierra)	1 oz.	1.3
Romano, grated:		
(Frigo)	1 T.	.2
(Kraft)	1 oz.	1.0
(Kraft) & parmesan	1 oz.	1.0
Roquefort (Kraft)	1 oz.	.5
Scamorze (Frigo)	1 oz.	.3
Swiss, domestic:		
Natural (Borden; Kraft; Sealtest)	1 oz.	.5
Process (Borden)	¾-oz. slice	.8
Swiss, imported, Finland or Switzerland (Borden)	1 oz.	.5
CHEESE FONDUE, *Swiss Knight*	1 oz. serving	1.0
CHEESE FOOD:		
American or cheddar:		
(Pauly)	.8-oz. slice	1.6
(Weight Watchers) colored or white	1-oz. slice	1.0

24

Food and Description	Measure or Quantity	Carbohydrates (grams)
Wispride, cheddar:		
Regular	1 oz.	7.0
& blue cheese	1 oz.	2.0
& port wine	1 oz.	2.0
& swiss cheese	1 oz.	7.0
Cheez 'n bacon, slices (Kraft)	¾-oz. slice	.8
Cheez 'n Crackers (Kraft)	1 piece	9.3
Cheez-ola (Fisher)	1 oz.	.5
Pimiento (Borden)	1 oz.	2.0
Pimiento (Pauly)	.8-oz. slice	.8
Swiss:		
(Borden) Cold-pack	.7-oz. slice	11.1
(Pauly)	.8-oz. slice	1.6
CHEESE PUFF, frozen (Durkee)	1 piece	3.0
CHEESE SPREAD:		
American or cheddar:		
(Borden)	.7-oz.	1.5
(Fisher)	1 oz.	2.0
(Nabisco) *Snack Mate*	1 tsp.	.3
(Pauly)	.8-oz.	1.2
Wispride, sharp	1 oz.	2.0
Bacon 'n Cheese (Borden)	1 oz.	1.8
Cheese 'n Bacon (Nabisco) *Snack Mate*	1 tsp.	.3
Cheez Whiz (Kraft)	1 oz.	1.8
Count Down (Fisher)	1 oz.	3.0
Garlic:		
(Borden)	1 oz.	1.8
(Kraft) *Squeeze-a-Snak*	1 oz.	.5
Imitation:		
(Fisher) *Chef's Delight*	1 oz.	3.0
(Kraft) *Calorie-Wise*	1 oz.	3.6
Limburger (Kraft)	1 oz.	.4
Neufchatel:		
Bacon & horseradish (Kraft) *Party Snack*	1 oz.	.7
Chipped beef, clam or pimiento (Kraft) *Party Snack*	1 oz.	1.2
Pineapple (Borden)	1 T.	1.8
Pimiento (Nabisco) *Snack Mate*	1 tsp.	1.8
Sharp (Pauly)	.8-oz.	.9
Smoke (Kraft) *Squeeze-a-Snak*	1 oz.	4.8
Swiss, process (Pauly)	.8-oz.	1.2
CHEESE STRAW, frozen (Durkee)	1 piece	1.0
CHELOIS WINE (Great Western)	3 fl. oz.	2.2
CHENIN BLANC WINE (Inglenook)	3 fl. oz.	1.3
CHERRY, sweet:		
Fresh, with stems	½ cup	10.2
Canned:		
(Stokely-Van Camp) solids & liq., pitted	½ cup	11.0

Food and Description	Measure or Quantity	Carbohydrates (grams)
(Del Monte) Royal Anne, solids & liq.	½ cup	26.8
Dietetic (Diet Delight) with pits, water pack, solids & liq.	½ cup	16.9
CHERRY, BLACK, SYRUP, dietetic (No-Cal)	1 tsp.	0
CHERRY BRANDY (DeKuyper)	1 fl. oz.	6.9
CHERRY, CANDIED	1 oz.	24.6
CHERRY DRINK:		
(Ann Page)	1 cup	30.9
(Hi-C)	6 fl. oz.	23.0
*Mix (Hi-C)	6 fl. oz.	19.0
CHERRY HEERING (Hiram Walker)	1 fl. oz.	10.0
CHERRY JELLY:		
Sweetened (Smucker's)	1 T.	13.5
Dietetic:		
(Featherweight)	1 T.	4.0
(Featherweight) artificially sweetened	1 T.	2.0
CHERRY LIQUEUR (DeKuyper)	1 fl. oz.	8.5
CHERRY, MARASCHINO (Liberty)	1 average cherry	1.9
CHERRY PRESERVE:		
Sweetened (Smucker's)	1 T.	13.5
Dietetic (Dia-Mel)	1 tsp.	0
CHERRY TURNOVER (Pillsbury)	1 turnover	25.0
CHESTNUT, fresh, in shell	¼ lb.	38.6
CHEWING GUM:		
Sweetened:		
Bazooka, bubble	1¢ slice	4.5
Beechies; Chiclets, tiny size	1 piece	1.6
Beech Nut; Beeman's; Big Red; Black Jack; Clove; Double-mint; Freedent; Fruit Punch; Juicy Fruit; Peppermint or sour lemon (Clark); *Spearmint* (Wrigley's); *Teaberry*	1 stick	2.3
Dentyne	1 piece	1.2
Dietetic:		
Bazooka sugarless	1 piece	Tr.
(Clark; *Care *Free*)	1 piece	1.7
(Estee; *Sug'r Like*)	1 piece	.6
CHIANTI WINE:		
(Antinori) Classico, or 1955 or vintage	3 fl. oz.	6.3
Brolio Classico	3 fl. oz.	.3
(Italian Swiss Colony)	3 fl. oz.	2.9
(Louis M. Martini)	3 fl. oz.	.2
CHICKARINA SOUP (Progresso)	1 cup	8.0
CHICKEN:		
Broiler, cooked, meat only	3 oz.	0
Fryer, fried, meat & skin	3 oz.	2.7

Food and Description	Measure or Quantity	Carbohydrates (grams)
Fryer, fried, meat only	3 oz.	1.0
Fryer, fried, a 2½-pound chicken (weighed with bone before cooking) will give you:		
Back	1 back	2.7
Breast	½ breast	1.1
Leg or drumstick	1 leg	.4
Neck	1 neck	1.9
Rib	1 rib	.8
Thigh	1 thigh	1.2
Wing	1 wing	.8
Fried skin	1 oz.	2.6
Hen & cock:		
Stewed, meat & skin	3 oz.	0
Stewed, dark meat only	3 oz.	0
Stewed, light meat only	3 oz.	0
Stewed, diced	½ cup	0
Roaster, roasted, dark or light meat without skin	3 oz.	0
CHICKEN A LA KING:		
Home recipe	1 cup	12.3
Canned:		
(Richardson & Robbins)	1 cup	14.4
(Swanson)	½ of 10½-oz. can	9.0
Frozen:		
(Banquet)	5-oz. bag	10.4
(Green Giant) *Toast Topper*	5-oz. pkg.	7.7
CHICKEN BOUILLON:		
(Cellu) low sodium	1 tsp.	2.0
(Croyden House)	1 tsp.	2.5
(Herb-Ox)	1 cube	.6
(Herb-Ox) instant	1 packet	1.9
(Maggi)	1 cube	1.0
MBT	1 packet	2.0
(Steero)	1 cube	.4
(Wyler's) instant	1 packet	.9
(Wyler's) no salt added	1 cube	1.6
CHICKEN CANNED, boned:		
(Lynden Farms) solids & liq.	5-oz. jar	0
(Swanson) with broth	5-oz. can	0
CHICKEN CROQUETTE DINNER, frozen (Morton)	10¼-oz. dinner	46.5
CHICKEN DINNER or LUNCHEON:		
Canned:		
(Lynden Farms) noodle with vegetables	½ of 15-oz. can	19.1
(Swanson) & dumplings	7½-oz. can	18.0
Frozen:		
(Banquet) & dumplings	2-lb. buffet bag	128.2
(Banquet) & dumplings	12-oz. dinner	36.4
(Banquet) *Man Pleaser*	17-oz. dinner	89.2

Food and Description	Measure or Quantity	Carbohydrates (grams)
(Green Giant) & biscuits	7-oz. serving	18.7
(Morton):		
Boneless	10-oz. dinner	22.8
Country Table	15-oz. dinner	94.8
& dumplings	11-oz. dinner	31.2
Fried	11-oz. dinner	50.0
& noodles	10¼-oz. dinner	40.8
(Swanson):		
Boneless, *Hungry Man*	19-oz. dinner	74.0
Fried	11½-oz. dinner	28.0
Fried, *Hungry Man*	15¾-oz. dinner	78.0
Fried, 3-course	15-oz. dinner	64.0
& noodles	10¼-oz. dinner	53.0
(Weight Watchers):		
Creole, casserole	13-oz. meal	11.8
Divan	9-oz. meal	7.9
with liver & onion	10½-oz. meal	11.0
Oriental-style	15-oz. meal	32.0
with stuffing	16-oz. meal	36.8
white meat	9-oz. meal	13.0
CHICKEN ENTREE, frozen:		
(Morton) fried, *Country Table*	12-oz. entree	27.3
(Green Giant) & biscuits, *Bake 'n Serve*	7-oz. entree	19.0
(Green Giant) and noodles, boil-in-bag	9-oz. bag	24.0
CHICKEN FRICASSE, canned		
(Richardson & Robbins)	1 cup	15.1
CHICKEN, FRIED:		
(Banquet)	11-oz. dinner	48.4
(Banquet)	2-lb. pkg.	117.3
(Swanson):		
Assorted pieces	1-lb. pkg.	40.0
Breast	3.2 oz.	8.0
Nibbles	3.2 oz.	12.0
Thighs & drumsticks	3.2 oz.	7.0
CHICKEN LIVER PUFF, frozen		
(Durkee)	½-oz. piece	3.0
CHICKEN & NOODLES:		
Canned (College Inn)	5-oz. serving	17.0
Frozen:		
(Banquet) buffet	2 lb.	79.1
(Green Giant)	9-oz. pkg.	21.5
CHICKEN PARMIGIANA, frozen		
(Weight Watchers)	9-oz. meal	8.9
CHICKEN PIE, frozen:		
(Banquet)	8-oz. pie	39.0
(Morton)	8-oz. pie	31.9
(Swanson)	8-oz. pie	44.0
(Swanson) *Hungry Man*	1-lb. pie	66.0
(Van de Kamp's)	7½-oz. pie	47.0
CHICKEN PUFF (Durkee)	½-oz. piece	3.0

28

Food and Description	Measure or Quantity	Carbohydrates (grams)
CHICKEN SALAD (Carnation)	1½ oz.	2.6
CHICKEN SOUP:		
Canned:		
*(Ann Page):		
Cream of	1 cup	9.3
& noodle	1 cup	8.7
& rice	1 cup	1.4
& stars	1 cup	7.4
& vegetables	1 cup	8.6
(Campbell):		
*Broth	8 oz.	2.4
Chunky	10¾-oz. can	22.0
Chunky, low sodium	7½-oz. can	13.0
*Cream of	8 oz.	8.0
*& dumplings	8 oz.	5.6
*Gumbo	8 oz.	8.0
Soup for One	7¾-oz. can	14.0
Noodle-O's	8 oz.	9.6
& rice, *Chunky*	19-oz. can	32.0
*& rice, condensed	8 oz.	5.6
*with stars	8 oz.	7.2
*& vegetables	8 oz.	8.6
Chunky	10¾-oz. can	25.0
(College Inn) broth	1 cup	.1
(Richardson & Robbins)	1 cup	1.6
(Swanson)	13¾-oz. can	4.0
Dietetic:		
*(Dia-Mel) & noodle	8 oz.	7.0
(Featherweight) & noodle, low sodium	8-oz. can	16.0
(Slim-ette) broth	8-oz. can	1.0
Mix:		
(Ann Page) & noodle	2-oz. pkg.	28.6
*(Lipton):		
Broth, *Cup-a-Broth*	6 fl. oz.	3.0
Cream of, *Cup-a-Soup*	1 pkg.	10.0
Giggle Noodle	1 cup (8 fl. oz.)	12.0
& noodle, with meat	1 cup (8 fl. oz.)	9.0
& rice	1 cup (8 fl. oz.)	8.0
& vegetables, *Cup-a-Soup*	6 fl. oz.	7.0
*(Nestlé's) *Souptime,* cream of	6 fl. oz.	8.0
*(Nestlé's) *Souptime,* & noodle	6 fl. oz.	4.0
*(Wyler's) cream of	1 pkg.	14.7
CHICKEN SPREAD:		
(Swanson)	5-oz. can	5.0
(Underwood)	1 oz.	1.1
CHICKEN STEW, canned:		
Regular pack:		
(B&M)	1 cup	15.3
(Bounty)	7½-oz. can	17.5
(Libby's) with dumplings	8 oz.	20.2

Food and Description	Measure or Quantity	Carbohydrates (grams)
(Swanson)	½ of 15¼-oz. can	18.2
Dietetic:		
(Dia-Mel)	8-oz. can	19.0
(Featherweight)	7¼-oz. can	21.0
CHICKEN TAMALE PIE		
(Lynden Farms)	½ tamale pie	12.0
CHICORY, WITLOOF, cut	½ cup	.8
CHILI or CHILI CON CARNE:		
Canned with beans:		
(Armour Star)	½ of 15½-oz. can	29.6
(Bounty)	7¾-oz. can	29.3
(Campbell) low sodium	7¾ oz.	30.0
(Hormel)	7½ oz.	23.6
(Libby's)	7½ oz.	32.2
(Morton House)	7½ oz.	27.0
(Rosarita)	8 oz.	27.2
(Swanson)	½ of 15½-oz. can	28.0
Dietetic (Featherweight)	8-oz. can	26.0
Canned without beans:		
(Armour Star)	½ of 15½-oz. can	22.7
(Hormel)	7½ oz.	7.6
(Libby's)	7½ oz.	32.2
(Morton House)	½ of 15-oz. can	14.0
CHILI BEEF SOUP:		
(Campbell) *Chunky*	11-oz. can	37.0
*(Campbell) condensed	8 oz.	19.2
CHILI SAUCE:		
(Hunt's)	1 T.	4.9
(Ortega) green	1 oz.	1.2
Dietetic (Featherweight)	1 T.	1.5
CHILI SEASONING MIX:		
(Ann Page)	1¾-oz. pkg.	29.8
*(Durkee)	1 cup	31.3
(French's) *Chili-O*	1 pkg.	23.6
CHINESE DINNER:		
Beef chop suey (Chun King)	11-oz. dinner	46.0
Chicken chow mein (Banquet)	12-oz. dinner	38.8
CHITTERLINGS (Hormel)	1-lb. 2-oz. can	.5
CHOCOLATE, BAKING (Hershey's):		
Bitter	1 oz.	6.8
Chips, dark	1 oz.	17.8
Chips, milk	1 oz.	18.2
CHOCOLATE DRINK:		
(Borden)	9½-fl.-oz. can	36.7
(Sealtest)	8 fl. oz.	24.0
CHOCOLATE DRINK MIX:		
(Borden) Dutch, instant	2 heaping tsps.	18.9
(Nestlé's) *Quik*	2 heaping tsps.	14.4
CHOCOLATE, HOT, home recipe	1 cup	26.0
CHOCOLATE ICE CREAM:		
(Borden) 9.5% fat	¼ pt.	16.9
(Prestige) French	¼ pt.	18.0

Food and Description	Measure or Quantity	Carbohydrates (grams)
(Sealtest)	¼ pt.	17.0
(Swift's)	½ cup	15.8
CHOCOLATE SYRUP:		
Sweetened:		
(Hershey's)	1 T.	8.3
Milk Mate	1½ T.	18.0
Dietetic:		
(Dia-Mel)	1 T.	3.3
(No-Cal)	1 tsp.	0
CHOP SUEY:		
Canned (Hung's):		
Chicken	8 oz.	12.3
Meatless	8 oz.	11.2
Frozen:		
(Banquet)	12-oz. dinner	38.8
(Banquet) beef	7-oz. bag	9.5
Mix:		
(Durkee)	1⅝-oz. pkg.	19.0
*(Durkee)	1 cup	12.0
CHOW MEIN:		
Canned:		
(Chun King):		
Beef	1 cup	11.0
Chicken	1 cup	11.2
Pork, *Divider-Pak*	7-oz. serving	11.0
(La Choy):		
Beef	1 cup	5.7
*Beef, bi-pack	1 cup	10.3
Chicken	¼ of 1-lb. can	5.0
*Chicken, bi-pack	1 cup	9.3
Meatless	1 cup	5.9
*Mushroom, bi-pack	1 cup	10.7
Pepper Oriental	1 cup	10.2
*Pepper Oriental, bi-pack	1 cup	11.1
*Pork, bi-pack	1 cup	10.6
Shrimp	1 cup	5.7
*Shrimp, bi-pack	1 cup	9.7
Frozen:		
(Banquet) chicken	7-oz. bag	9.7
(Green Giant) chicken	9-oz. entree	15.0
(La Choy):		
Beef dinner, 5-compartment	11-oz. dinner	52.8
Chicken dinner	11-oz. dinner	53.8
Chicken entree	8-oz. serving	9.1
Pepper Oriental dinner	11-oz. dinner	54.6
Pepper Oriental entree	7½-oz. serving	11.5
Shrimp dinner	11-oz. dinner	55.4
Shrimp entree	8-oz. serving	10.9
(Temple) shrimp	1 cup	15.0
CHUTNEY (Major Grey's)	1 T.	13.1
CINNAMON, ground (French's)	1 tsp.	1.4

Food and Description	Measure or Quantity	Carbohydrates (grams)
CITRUS COOLER:		
(Ann Page)	1 cup	29.4
(Hi-C)	6 fl. oz.	23.0
CLAM:		
Raw, all kinds, meat only	1 cup (8 oz.)	13.4
Raw, soft, meat & liq.	1 lb. (weighed in shell)	5.3
Canned:		
(Doxsee) chopped & minced, solids & liq.	4 oz.	3.2
(Doxsee) chopped, meat only	4 oz.	2.1
Frozen (Mrs. Paul's):		
Deviled	3-oz. piece	14.4
Fried	½ of 5-oz. pkg.	24.1
CLAMATO COCKTAIL (Mott's)	6 fl. oz.	19.0
CLAM CAKE, thins (Mrs. Paul's)	2½-oz. piece	16.6
CLAM CHOWDER, canned:		
Manhattan:		
*(Campbell)	8 oz.	12.0
(Campbell) *Chunky*	½ of 19-oz. can	23.0
(Crosse & Blackwell)	½ of 13-oz. can	9.0
(Progresso)	1 cup	16.0
(Snow)	8 oz.	10.4
New England:		
*(Campbell)	8 oz.	10.4
(Crosse & Blackwell)	½ of 13-oz. can	14.0
(Doxsee)	1 cup	27.0
CLAM COCKTAIL (Sau-Sea)	4-oz. jar	19.1
CLAM FRITTERS	2" x 1¾" fritter	12.4
CLAM JUICE (Snow)	½ cup	1.2
CLAM SOUP MIX (Wyler's)	1 pkg.	12.6
CLAM STICK, breaded (Mrs. Paul's)	8-oz. piece	6.5
CLARET WINE:		
(Gold Seal)	3 fl. oz.	.4
(Inglenook) Navelle	3 fl. oz.	.3
(Taylor) 12.5% alcohol	3 fl. oz.	2.4
CLORETS, gum or mint	1 piece	1.3
CLOVES (French's)	1 tsp.	1.2
COCKTAIL HOST MIX (Holland House)	1½ fl. oz.	18.0
COCOA:		
Dry, unsweetened:		
(Droste)	1 T.	2.9
(Hershey's)	1 T.	3.3
(Sultana)	1 T.	3.5
Mix:		
(Alba '66) instant	1 envelope	10.2
(Alba '66) chocolate & marshmallow flavor	1 envelope	10.0
(Carnation) all flavors	1-oz. pkg.	22.0
(Hershey's) hot	1 oz.	21.0

32

Food and Description	Measure or Quantity	Carbohydrates (grams)
(Hershey's) instant	3 T.	17.0
(Nestlé) hot	1 oz.	22.0
(Nestlé) with mini marshmallows	1 oz.	23.0
(Ovaltine) hot	1-oz. pkg.	22.0
Swiss Miss	1 oz.	21.0
Swiss Miss, instant, double rich	1 oz.	20.0
Swiss Miss, instant, with mini marshmallows	1.1 oz.	22.0
Dietetic:		
(Ovaltine) hot	.7-oz. pkg.	15.0
Swiss Miss, instant, lite	3 T.	17.0
COCOA KRISPIES, cereal	¾ cup	26.0
COCOA PUFFS, cereal	1 oz.	25.0
COCONUT:		
Fresh, meat only	2" x 2" x ½" piece	4.2
Grated or shredded, loosely packed	½ cup	6.1
Dried:		
(Baker's) *Angel Flake*	¼ cup	7.9
(Baker's) cookie	¼ cup	12.2
(Baker's) premium shred	¼ cup	9.0
(Durkee) shredded	¼ cup	2.0
COCO WHEATS, cereal	3 T.	28.5
COD, broiled	3 oz.	0
COFFEE:		
Regular:		
*(*Max-Pax;* Maxwell House; Maxwell House Electra Perk; Yuban; *Yuban Electra Matic*)	6 fl. oz.	0
**Mellow Roast*	6 fl. oz.	2.0
Decaffeinated:		
**Brim,* regular or electric perk	6 fl. oz.	0
**Brim,* freeze-dried	6 fl. oz.	1.0
Decaf	1 tsp.	1.0
Nescafé, freeze-dried	1 rounded tsp.	1.0
**Sanka,* regular or electric perk	6 fl. oz.	0
**Sanka,* freeze-dried or instant	6 fl. oz.	1.0
**Freeze-dried:*		
(*Maxim; Sanka; Taster's Choice*)	6 fl. oz.	1.0
Instant:		
(Borden; *Kava*)	1 rounded tsp.	.9
*(Chase & Sanborn)	5 fl. oz.	Tr.
**Mellow Roast*	6 fl. oz.	2.0
Nescafé	1 slightly rounded tsp.	1.0
*(Sanka; Maxwell House)	6 fl. oz.	1.0
**Mix (General Foods):		
Café Français, Cafe Vienna, Irish Mocha Mint, Orange Cappuccino, Suisse Mocha	6 fl. oz.	7.0
COFFEE CAKE (See CAKE, Coffee)		
COFFEE ICE CREAM (Breyer's)	¼ pt.	15.0

33

Food and Description	Measure or Quantity	Carbohydrates (grams)
COFFEE SOUTHERN	1 fl. oz.	8.8
COFFEE SYRUP (No-Cal)	1 tsp.	.4
COLA SOFT DRINK (See SOFT DRINK, Cola)		
COLA SYRUP (No-Cal)	1 tsp.	Tr.
COLD DUCK WINE (Great Western) pink	3 fl. oz.	7.7
COLESLAW, not drained, made with mayonnaise-type salad dressing	1 cup	8.5
COLLARDS:		
Leaves, cooked	½ cup	4.8
Frozen (Birds Eye) chopped	⅓ pkg.	4.0
COLLINS MIX (Bar-Tender's)	1 serving	17.4
CONCENTRATE, cereal	⅓ cup	15.0
CONCORD WINE:		
(Gold Seal)	3 fl. oz.	9.8
(Mogen David)	3 fl. oz.	16.0
CONSOMMÉ MADRILENE (Crosse & Blackwell):		
Clear	½ of 13-oz. can	4.0
Red	½ of 13-oz. can	0
COOKIE:		
Almond toast	1 piece	9.6
Animal cracker:		
(Keebler)	1 piece	1.9
(Nabisco) Barnum's Animals	1 piece	1.9
(Sunshine)	1 piece	1.7
Anisette sponge (Stella D'oro)	1 piece	10.0
Anisette toast (Stella D'oro)	1 piece	7.8
Arrowroot (Sunshine)	1 piece	3.0
Assortment:		
(Stella D'oro) Lady Stella	1 piece	5.0
(Sunshine) Lady Joan	1 piece	5.8
(Sunshine) Lady Joan, iced	1 piece	6.1
Aunt Sally, iced (Sunshine)	1 piece	19.7
Big Treat (Sunshine)	1 piece	26.6
Biscos (Nabisco) waffle creme	1 piece	6.0
Bordeaux (Pepperidge Farm)	1 piece	5.1
Breakfast Treats (Stella D'oro)	1 piece	15.5
Brown edge wafers (Nabisco)	1 piece	4.2
Brownie:		
(Drake's) Junior	⅔-oz. cake	10.0
(Frito-Lays) nut fudge	1.8-oz. piece	34.0
(Hostess) 2 to pkg.	1¼-oz. piece	24.1
(Pepperidge Farm) nut	1 piece	6.3
(Tastykake)	1 pkg.	34.0
(Tastykake) peanut butter	1 pkg.	32.0
Brussels (Pepperidge Farm)	1 piece	4.6
Butter (Nabisco; Sunshine)	1 piece	3.3
Buttercup (Keebler)	1 piece	3.6
Butterscotch Fudgies (Tastykake)	1 pkg.	35.0
Capri (Pepperidge Farm)	1 piece	9.7

34

Food and Description	Measure or Quantity	Carbohydrates (grams)
Cardiff (Pepperidge Farm)	1 piece	2.5
Cheda-Nut (Nabisco)	1 piece	4.5
Cherry Coolers (Sunshine)	1 piece	4.5
Chocolate & chocolate-covered:		
Pinwheels (Nabisco)	1 piece	21.0
Snaps (Sunshine)	1 piece	2.4
Wafers (Nabisco) Famous	1 piece	4.8
Chocolate chip:		
(Drake's)	1 piece	9.9
(Keebler):		
C. C. Biggs	1 piece	6.9
100's	1 piece	3.3
Rich 'N Chips	1 piece	10.0
(Nabisco) Chips Ahoy	1 piece	7.3
(Pepperidge Farm)	1 piece	6.2
(Sunshine) Chip-a-Roo's	1 piece	7.7
(Tastykake) Choc-o-Chip	1¾-oz. pk.	34.8
Cinnamon:		
(Pepperidge Farm) sugar	1 piece	7.0
(Sunshine) toast	1 piece	2.3
Coconut:		
(Keebler) chocolate drop	1 piece	9.4
(Nabisco) bar	1 piece	6.3
(Sunshine) bar	1 piece	6.2
(Sunshine) chocolate chip	1 piece	9.7
(Tastykake) coconut kiss	1 piece	8.3
Cream Lunch (Sunshine)	1 piece	7.3
Creme wafer stick (Dutch Twin)	1 piece	5.9
Creme wafer stick (Nabisco)	1 piece	6.0
Devil's food cake (Nabisco)	1 piece	10.5
Dixie Vanilla (Sunshine)	1 piece	13.1
Dresden (Pepperidge Farm)	1 piece	10.0
Egg Jumbo (Stella D'oro)	1 piece	7.6
Fig bar:		
(Keebler)	1 piece	13.0
(Nabisco) Fig Newtons	1 piece	11.5
(Sunshine)	1 piece	9.2
Fudge:		
(Keebler) fudge stripes	1 piece	7.3
(Pepperidge Farm) chips	1 piece	6.7
(Planters) creme	1 oz.	20.0
(Sunshine)	1 piece	9.4
Gingersnap:		
(Nabisco) old fashioned	1 piece	5.5
(Sunshine)	1 piece	4.4
Golden Bars (Stella D'oro)	1 piece	6.0
Golden Fruit (Sunshine)	1 piece	14.4
Hermit bar, frosted (Tastykake)	1 pkg.	60.8
Hostest with the Mostest (Stella D'oro)	1 piece	5.2
Hydrox (Sunshine):		
Regular or mint	1 piece	7.1

Food and Description	Measure or Quantity	Carbohydrates (grams)
Vanilla	1 piece	7.1
Ladyfinger	3¼" x 1⅜" x 1⅛"	7.1
Lemon:		
(Sunshine)	1 piece	9.8
(Planters) Creme	1 oz.	20.0
(Pepperidge Farm) nut crunch	1 piece	6.4
(Sunshine) lemon Coolers	1 piece	4.5
Lido (Pepperidge Farm)	1 piece	10.0
Lisbon (Pepperidge)	1 piece	3.3
Macaroon:		
Almond (Tastykake)	1 piece	17.5
Coconut (Nabisco) *Bake Shop*	1 piece	12.4
Fudge (Hostess)	1 piece	32.7
Margherite (Stella D'oro)	1 piece	10.6
Marquisette (Pepperidge Farm)	1 piece	5.0
Marshmallow:		
Banana pie (Planters)	1 oz.	22.0
Chocolate pie (Planters)	1 oz.	22.0
Mallowmars (Nabisco)	1 piece	9.0
Mallow Puff (Sunshine)	1 piece	12.2
Puffs (Nabisco) chocolate-coated	1 piece	13.0
Sandwich (Nabisco)	1 piece	6.0
Milano (Pepperidge Farm)	1 piece	7.2
Milano, mint (Pepperidge Farm)	1 piece	8.4
Mint sandwich (Nabisco) *Mystic*	1 piece	10.6
Molasses	1 oz.	21.5
Molasses & spice (Sunshine)	1 piece	11.9
Naples (Pepperidge Farm)	1 piece	3.7
Nassau (Pepperidge Farm)	1 piece	9.2
Oatmeal:		
(Drake's)	1 piece	10.1
(Nabisco)	1 piece	11.5
(Nabisco) raisin, *Bake Shop*	1 piece	11.5
(Pepperidge Farm) Irish	1 piece	7.1
(Pepperidge Farm) raisin	1 piece	7.5
(Sunshine) iced	1 piece	11.6
(Sunshine) peanut butter	1 piece	10.5
(Tastykake) raisin bar	1 pkg.	47.6
Old Country Treats (Stella D'oro)	1 piece	7.1
Orleans (Pepperidge Farm)	1 piece	2.5
Peanut & peanut butter:		
(Nabisco) creme patties	1 piece	4.0
(Nabisco) sandwich, *Nutter Butter*	1 piece	9.5
(Sunshine) patties	1 piece	4.2
Pecan Sandies (Keebler)	1 piece	9.4
Pirouette (Pepperidge Farm)	1 piece	4.5
Pitter Patter (Keebler)	1 piece	11.0
Pizelle (Stella D'oro)	1 piece	6.7
Raisin	1 oz.	22.9
Raisin, fruit biscuit (Nabisco)	1 piece	12.0

Food and Description	Measure or Quantity	Carbohydrates (grams)
Sandwich, creme:		
(Keebler):		
Chocolate fudge	1 piece	12.0
Coconut fruit	1 piece	8.3
Elfwich	1 piece	7.8
Lemon fruit	1 piece	8.3
Orange fruit	1 piece	8.3
Pitter Patter	1 piece	11.0
Vanilla, French	1 piece	12.0
(Nabisco):		
Cameo	1 piece	10.5
Assorted *Cookie Break*	1 piece	7.3
Vanilla Cookie Break	1 piece	7.3
Oreo	1 piece	7.3
Oreo, Double Stuf	1 piece	9.0
Oreo & Swiss, assortment	1 piece	7.0
Social Tea	1 piece	3.5
Swiss	1 piece	7.7
(Sunshine):		
Obit	1 piece	7.0
Vienna Finger	1 piece	10.5
Sesame, *Regina* (Stella D'oro)	1 piece	6.9
Shortbread or shortcake:		
(Pepperidge Farm)	1 piece	8.3
Lorna Doone (Nabisco)	1 piece	4.8
Pecan (Nabisco)	1 piece	8.5
Scotties (Sunshine)	1 piece	5.0
Social Tea Biscuit (Nabisco)	1 piece	3.5
Spiced wafers (Nabisco)	1 piece	5.8
Sprinkles (Sunshine)	1 piece	11.4
Sugar cookies:		
(Nabisco) rings	1 piece	10.5
(Pepperidge Farm)	1 piece	7.0
(Pepperidge Farm) brown	1 piece	6.9
Sugar wafer:		
(Dutch Treat)	1 piece	6.3
(Dutch Twin)	1 piece	6.2
(Keebler) *Krisp Kreem*	1 piece	4.2
(Nabisco) *Biscos*	1 piece	2.5
(Sunshine) lemon	1 piece	6.5
Tahiti (Pepperidge Farm)	1 piece	8.6
Toy (Sunshine)	1 piece	2.1
Vanilla creme (Wise)	1 piece	5.0
Vanilla creme (Planters)	1 oz.	20.0
Vanilla wafer:		
(Keebler; Nabisco *Nilla*)	1 piece	2.6
(Sunshine) small	1 piece	2.2
Venice (Pepperidge Farm)	1 piece	6.3
Waffle creme (Dutch Twin)	1 piece	5.7
Yum Yums (Sunshine)	1 piece	10.4
COOKIE, DIETETIC:		
Angel puffs (Stella D'oro)	1 piece	1.5

Food and Description	Measure or Quantity	Carbohydrates (grams)
Assorted (Estee)	1 piece	3.0
Bittersweet chocolate wafer (Estee)	1 piece	10.0
Chocolate chip (Estee)	1 piece	4.0
Chocolate chip, *Sug'r Like*	1 piece	4.0
Chocolate flavored bar, *Sug'r Like*	1 piece	4.0
Chocolate crescent, *Sug'r Like*	1 piece	4.0
Chocolate wafer (Estee)	1 piece	2.4
Chocolate wafer, *Sug'r Like*	1 piece	4.0
Duplex, *Sug'r Like*	1 piece	6.0
Fig pastry (Stella D'oro)	1 piece	15.5
Fruit wafer (Estee)	1 piece	2.7
Kichel (Stella D'oro)	1 piece	.7
Lemon, *Sug'r Like*	1 piece	4.0
Lemon thin (Estee)	1 piece	4.0
Milk chocolate wafer (Estee)	1 piece	10.0
Oatmeal raisin (Estee)	1 piece	4.0
Peanut butter creme wafer, *Sug'r Like*	1 piece	3.0
Prune pastry (Stella D'oro)	1 piece	14.3
Rich crisp bar, *Sug'r Like*	1 piece	4.5
Sandwich (Estee)	1 piece	8.0
Sandwich (Estee) lemon	1 piece	8.0
Vanilla, *Sug'r Like*	1 piece	4.0
Vanilla thin (Estee)	1 piece	4.0
Vanilla wafer, *Sug'r Like*	1 piece	4.0
Wafer (Estee) assorted	1 piece	4.1
COOKIE CRISP, cereal:		
Chocolate chip and vanilla wafer	1 cup	25.0
Oatmeal	1 cup	24.0
*****COOKIE DOUGH** (Pillsbury):		
Butterscotch nut	1 cookie	6.7
Chocolate chip	1 cookie	7.3
Oatmeal & chocolate chip	1 cookie	7.3
Oatmeal raisin	1 cookie	8.7
Peanut butter	1 cookie	6.3
Sugar	1 cookie	8.3
COOKIE MIX:		
*Brownie (Betty Crocker):		
Fudge	⅟₁₆ of pan	21.0
German chocolate	⅟₁₆ of pan	26.0
*Date bar (Betty Crocker)	⅟₃₂ of pkg.	9.0
*Macaroon, coconut (Betty Crocker)	⅟₂₄ of pkg.	10.0
*Peanut butter (Quaker)	1 cookie	8.0
*Pecan bar (Pillsbury)	2" x 1¼"	10.5
*Sugar (Quaker)	1 cookie	9.5
*Dietetic (Dia-Mel)	2" cookie	7.0
COOKING SPRAY, *Mazola No Stick*	2-second spray	0
CORIANDER, seed (French's)	1 tsp.	.8
CORN:		
Fresh, on the cob, boiled	5" x 1¾" ear	16.2

Food and Description	Measure or Quantity	Carbohydrates (grams)
Canned, regular pack:		
(Del Monte):		
Cream style	½ cup	22.2
Whole kernel, drained	½ cup	21.3
Whole kernel, vacuum pack	½ cup	21.6
(Green Giant):		
Cream style	4¼ oz.	22.3
Whole kernel, solids & liq.	4¼-oz. serving	15.8
Whole kernel, *Mexicorn,* solids & liq.	4-oz. serving	20.3
Whole kernel, *Niblets,* vacuum pack	4-oz. serving	19.5
(Le Sueur) solids & liq.	4¼ oz.	17.3
(Libby's):		
Cream style	½ cup	21.2
Whole kernel, solids & liq.	½ cup	18.8
(Stokely-Van Camp) whole kernel, solids & liq.	½ cup	17.6
Canned, dietetic pack:		
(Blue Boy) cream style	4 oz.	20.6
(Diet Delight) solids & liq.	½ cup	14.6
(Featherweight):		
Cream style	½ cup	18.0
Whole kernel, solids & liq.	½ cup	16.0
(Tillie Lewis) solids & liq.	½ cup	15.4
Frozen:		
(Birds Eye):		
On the cob	4.9-oz. ear	28.0
On the cob, *Little Ears*	1 ear	16.0
Whole kernel	⅓ of pkg.	18.0
(Green Giant):		
On the cob	5½" ear	32.7
On the cob, *Nibbler*	3" ear	18.0
Whole kernel, golden	4-oz. serving	20.5
Whole kernel, golden, in butter sauce, *Mexicorn* & *Niblets*	⅓ pkg.	14.2
Whole kernel, white, in butter sauce	⅓ pkg.	15.2
(Ore-Ida):		
On the cob	1 ear	27.0
Whole kernel	3.2-oz. serving	21.3
CORNBREAD:		
Home recipe:		
Corn pone	4 oz.	41.1
Spoon bread	4 oz.	19.2
*Mix:		
(Aunt Jemima)	⅙ of cornbread	34.0
(Dromedary)	2" x 2" piece	19.0
(Pillsbury) *Ballard*	1/16 of recipe	26.0
CORN CHEX, cereal	1 cup	25.0
CORN CHOWDER (Snow)	8 oz.	19.6

Food and Description	Measure or Quantity	Carbohydrates (grams)
CORNED BEEF:		
Cooked, boneless, medium fat	4 oz.	0
Canned:		
(Armour Star)	⅓ of 12-oz. can	0
(Hormel) *Dinty Moore*	4 oz.	0
(Libby's)	½ of 7-oz. can	1.9
(Wilson) brisket, *Tender Made*	4 oz.	1.0
Packaged:		
(Oscar Mayer) jellied loaf	1-oz. slice	0
(Vienna) brisket	1 oz.	0
(Vienna) flats	1 oz.	.1
CORNED BEEF HASH, canned:		
(A&P)	15-oz. can	39.8
(Bounty)	7½-oz. can	22.2
(Hormel) *Mary Kitchen*	7½-oz. can	21.0
(Libby's)	1 cup	31.1
CORNED BEEF HASH DINNER, frozen (Banquet)	10-oz. dinner	42.6
CORNED BEEF SPREAD		
(Underwood)	1 oz.	Tr.
CORN FLAKE CRUMBS (Kellogg's)	¼ cup	25.0
CORN FLAKES, cereal:		
(Featherweight) low sodium	1 oz.	25.0
(General Mills) *Country*	1 cup	24.0
(Kellogg's)	1 cup	25.0
(Post) *Post Toasties*	1¼ cups	24.4
(Ralston Purina)	1 cup	24.0
(Van Brode)	1 oz.	24.4
(Van Brode) low sodium	1 oz.	25.1
(Van Brode) sugar toasted	1 oz.	25.6
CORN FRITTER (Mrs. Paul's)	2-oz. fritter	15.4
CORN MEAL:		
Bolted (Aunt Jemima/Quaker)	3 T.	21.2
Degermed	¼ cup	27.5
Mix:		
Bolted (Aunt Jemima)	1 cup	80.4
Degermed (Aunt Jemima)	1 cup	84.0
CORNSTARCH (Argo; Kingsford's, Duryea's)	1 tsp.	2.7
CORN SYRUP	1 T.	15.8
CORN TOTAL, cereal (General Mills)	1 cup	24.0
CORNY-SNAPS, cereal (Kellogg's)	1 cup	24.0
COUGH DROP:		
(Beech-Nut)	1 drop	2.4
(H-B)	1 drop	1.9
(Luden's)	1 drop	2.1
(Pine Bros.)	1 drop	2.0
(Smith Brothers)	1 drop	2.1
COUNT CHOCULA, cereal (General Mills)	1 oz.	24.0
COUNTRY CHERRY, wine (Annie Green Springs) 9% alcohol	3 fl. oz.	6.8

Food and Description	Measure or Quantity	Carbohydrates (grams)
COUNTRY CRISP, cereal	¾ cup	24.4
COUNTRY MORNING, cereal (Kellogg's):		
Regular	⅓ cup	18.0
With raisins & dates	⅓ cup	19.0
CRAB:		
Fresh, steamed:		
Whole	½ lb.	.6
Meat only	4 oz.	.6
Canned, king crab (Icy Point; Pillar Rock)	½ of 7½-oz. can	1.1
Frozen (Wakefield's Alaska King)	4 oz.	.6
CRAB APPLE	¼ lb.	18.5
CRAB CAKE THINS, breaded & fried (Mrs. Paul's)	½ of 10-oz. pkg.	35.3
CRAB COCKTAIL (Sau-Sea)	4-oz. jar	18.4
CRAB DEVILED, breaded & fried (Mrs. Paul's)	½ of 6-oz. pkg.	18.3
CRAB IMPERIAL, home recipe	1 cup	8.6
CRAB SOUP (Crosse & Blackwell)	½ of 13-oz. can	8.0
CRACKERS. PUFFS & CHIPS:		
American Harvest (Nabisco)	1 piece	2.0
Arrowroot biscuit (Nabisco)	1 piece	3.5
Bacon-flavored thins (Nabisco)	1 piece	1.3
Bacon Nips	1 oz.	15.6
Bacon rinds (Wonder)	1 oz.	0
Bacon toast (Keebler)	1 piece	2.1
Bacon Tasters (Old London)	½-oz. bag	8.8
Bakon-Snacks	1 oz.	14.3
Betcha Bacon	1 oz.	18.0
Bugles (General Mills)	1 oz.	17.0
Butter thins (Nabisco)	1 piece	2.2
Cheese-flavored:		
Chedda Bitz (Frito-Lay)	1 oz.	18.9
Cheese balls (Planters)	1 oz.	4.3
Cheese 'n Cracker (Kraft)	4 crackers & ¾ oz. cheese	.7
Cheese curls (Planters)	1 oz.	4.3
Cheese Nips (Nabisco)	1 piece	.7
Cheese Pixies (Wise) baked	1-oz. bag	15.7
Cheese Pixies (Wise) fried	1 oz.	15.6
Cheese Shindig (Keebler)	1 piece	.9
Chee.Tos, baked	1 oz.	15.4
Chee.Tos, crunchy	1 oz.	15.4
Cheez Balls (Planters)	1 oz.	15.0
Cheez Curls (Planters)	1 oz.	15.0
Cheez Doodles (Old London) baked	½-oz. pkg.	7.9
Cheez Doodles (Old London) fried	1 oz.	15.6
Cheez-Its (Sunshine)	1 piece	.6
Cheez Waffles (Austin's)	1 piece	1.3

Food and Description	Measure or Quantity	Carbohydrates (grams)
Parmesan Swirl (Nabisco)	1 piece	1.2
Sandwich (Planters)	1 piece	3.0
Swiss cheese (Nabisco)	1 piece	1.1
Tid-Bits (Nabisco)	1 piece	.5
Twists (Bachman)	1 oz.	17.0
Twists (Wonder)	1 oz.	14.7
Chicken in a Biskit (Nabisco)	1 piece	1.1
Chipos (General Mills)	1 oz.	17.0
Chipsters (Nabisco)	1 piece	.3
Clam-flavored crisps (Snow)	1 oz.	14.9
Club Cracker (Keebler)	1 piece	2.1
Corn capers (Wonder)	1 oz.	15.4
Corn chips:		
(Bachman)	1 oz.	17.0
Cornetts	1 oz.	16.3
Dipsy Doodles (Old London)	1 oz.	15.5
Fritos	1 oz.	15.5
Korkers (Nabisco)	1 piece	.8
(Old London)	1-oz. bag	16.7
(Planters)	1 oz.	15.0
Corn Nuggets (Frito-Lay's)	1 oz.	21.2
Crown Pilot (Nabisco)	1 piece	12.5
Doo Dads (Nabisco)	1 piece	.3
Escort (Nabisco)	1 piece	2.7
Flings, cheese (Nabisco)	1 piece	.8
Goldfish (Pepperidge Farm)	5 pieces	1.6
Graham:		
(Keebler) honey	1 piece	3.0
(Nabisco)	1 piece	5.3
(Nabisco) Cinnamon Treat	1 piece	5.0
Graham, chocolate or cocoa-covered:		
(Keebler) Deluxe	1 piece	5.6
(Nabisco)	1 piece	7.0
(Nabisco) Fancy Dip	1 piece	8.5
Graham, sugar-honey coated		
(Nabisco) Honey Maid	1 piece	5.5
Hi-Ho (Sunshine)	1 piece	2.1
Hot Potatas (Old London)	⅝-oz. bag	12.0
Ideal Flatbrod:		
Caraway & whole grain	1 piece	4.0
Ultra thin	1 piece	3.0
Lil' Loaf (Nabisco)	1 stick	1.8
Matzo (See MATZO)		
Melba Toast (See MELBA)		
Milk Lunch (Keebler)	1 piece	4.5
Milk lunch (Nabisco) Royal Lunch	1 piece	7.9
Munchos	1 oz.	15.2
Onion-flavored:		
Funyuns (Frito-Lay)	1 oz.	18.9
(Keebler) toast	1 piece	2.1
(Nabisco) French	1 piece	1.5

Food and Description	Measure or Quantity	Carbohydrates (grams)
(Old London) rings	½-oz. bag	10.4
(Pepperidge Farm) thins	1 piece	2.0
(Snow) crisps	1 piece	15.9
(Wise) rings	½-oz. bag	11.1
(Wonder) rings	1 oz.	19.5
Oyster:		
(Keebler) *Zesta*	1 piece	.2
Dandy or *Oysterettes* (Nabisco)	1 piece	.6
(Sunshine) mini	1 piece	.6
Peanut butter 'n cheez crackers (Kraft)	4 crackers and ¾ oz. peanut butter	13.4
Peanut butter sandwich:		
(Planters) cheese crackers	1 piece	3.0
(Wise) cheese crackers	1 piece	3.4
(Wise) toasted crackers	1 piece	3.7
Pizza Wheels (Wise)	¾-oz. bag	16.1
Ritz (Nabisco)	1 piece	2.0
Roman Meal Wafers	1 piece	2.4
Ry-Krisp, natural	1 triple cracker	5.0
Ry-Krisp, seasoned	1 triple cracker	4.5
Rye, *Wasa-Crisp*:		
Golden	1 piece	8.0
Lite	1 piece	6.0
Seasoned	1 piece	7.0
Rye thins (Pepperidge Farm)	1 piece	2.0
Rye toast (Keebler)	1 piece	2.2
Rye wafers (Nabisco)	1 piece	4.5
Saltine:		
Flavor-Kist	1 piece	2.2
Hi-Ho (Sunshine)	1 piece	2.1
Krispy (Sunshine)	1 piece	2.0
Premium (Nabisco); *Zesta* (Keebler)	1 piece	2.0
Sesame:		
(Keebler) toast	1 piece	2.1
(Nabisco) buttery-flavored	1 piece	1.9
(Sunshine) *La Lanne*	1 piece	1.8
Sea Wheat (Austin's)	1 piece	3.7
Sociables (Nabisco)	1 piece	1.3
Soda (Sunshine)	1 piece	2.3
Star Lites (Wise)	1 cup	9.9
Taco corn chips (Old London; Wise)	1 oz.	20.0
Taco tortilla chips (Wonder)	1 oz.	15.9
Tortilla chips:		
(Bachman) nacho or taco flavor	1 oz.	17.0
Doritos, regular	1 oz.	18.3
Doritos, taco flavor	1 oz.	17.9
(Planters) nacho or taco flavor	1 oz.	14.0
Triscuit (Nabisco)	1 piece	3.0
Twigs (Nabisco)	1 stick	1.6

Food and Description	Measure or Quantity	Carbohydrates (grams)
Uneeda Biscuit (Nabisco)	1 piece	3.7
Unsalted crackers (Cellu)	1 piece	2.5
Wafer-ets (Hol-Grain):		
Rice	1 piece	2.5
Wheat	1 piece	2.5
Waldorf (Keebler) low sodium	1 piece	2.4
Waverly Wafer (Nabisco)	1 piece	2.6
Wheat chips (General Mills)	4 pieces	2.6
Wheat thins (Nabisco)	1 piece	1.2
Whistles (General Mills)	17 pieces	8.0
White thins (Pepperidge Farm)	1 piece	2.0
CRACKER CRUMBS, graham (Nabisco)	⅛ of 9″ pie shell	12.0
CRANAPPLE JUICE (Ocean Spray):		
Regular	6 fl. oz.	36.3
Low calorie	6 fl. oz.	7.8
CRANBERRY, fresh (Ocean Spray)	½ cup	23.9
CRANBERRY-APPLE DRINK (Ann Page)	½ cup	22.6
CRANBERRY JUICE COCKTAIL:		
(Ann Page)	½ cup	22.6
(Lincoln)	6 fl. oz.	28.5
(Ocean Spray):		
Regular	6 fl. oz.	27.0
Dietetic	6 fl. oz.	9.3
*Frozen	6 fl. oz.	28.3
CRANBERRY-ORANGE JUICE DRINK (Ocean Spray)	6 fl. oz.	24.6
CRANBERRY-ORANGE RELISH (Ocean Spray)	1 T.	8.2
CRANBERRY SAUCE:		
Home recipe	4 oz.	51.6
(Ocean Spray):		
Jellied	2 oz.	21.8
Whole berry	2 oz.	22.0
CRANBREAKER MIX (Bar-Tender's)	1 serving	17.4
CRANGRAPE (Ocean Spray)	6 fl. oz.	29.8
CRANICOT (Ocean Spray)	6 fl. oz.	32.8
CRANPRUNE JUICE (Ocean Spray)	6 fl. oz.	32.8
CRAZY BONE (Drake's)	1-oz. cake	18.6
CRAZY COW, cereal (General Mills)	1 cup	24.0
CREAM:		
Half & Half:		
(Dean)	1 T.	.7
10.5% fat (Sealtest)	1 T.	1.0
12.8% fat (Meadow Gold)	1 T.	.6
Light, table or coffee:		
16% fat (Sealtest)	1 T.	.6
18% fat (Sealtest)	1 T.	.6
Light whipping, 30% fat (Sealtest)	1 T.	1.0
Heavy whipping (Dean; Meadow Gold; Sealtest)	1 T.	.5

Food and Description	Measure or Quantity	Carbohydrates (grams)
Sour:		
(Axelrod)	¼ of 8-oz. container	2.2
(Borden; Breakstone; Dean)	1 T.	.6
Imitation:		
(Pet)	1 T.	1.0
Sour Slim (Dean)	1 T.	3.3
Sour Treat (Delite)	1 T.	.8
Sour dressing (Breakstone)	1 T.	.7
Substitute (See **CREAM SUBSTITUTE**)		
CREAM PUFFS:		
Custard filling, home recipe	3½" x 2"	26.7
***CREAM OF RICE**, cereal*	4 oz.	17.9
***CREAMSICLE** (Popsicle Industries)*	2½ fl. oz.	12.8
CREAM SUBSTITUTE:		
(Alba) *Dairy Light*	2.8-oz. envelope	1.0
Coffee-mate; Cremora; Pream	1 tsp.	1.1
Coffee Rich	½ oz.	2.1
Coffee Twin	½ fl. oz.	1.0
Half & Half (Meadow Gold)	1 T.	1.2
N-Rich	1 tsp.	1.7
Perx	1½ tsp.	.6
(Pet)	1 tsp.	1.0
Poly Perx	½ oz.	2.0
(Sanna)	1 plastic cup	2.0
***CREAM OF WHEAT**, cereal:*		
*Instant	¾ cup	21.0
Mix 'n Eat, dry:		
Regular	1 packet	21.0
Baked apple & cinnamon	1 packet	29.0
Banana & spice	1 packet	29.0
Maple & brown sugar	3¾ T.	29.0
Quick	2½ T.	21.0
Regular	2½ T.	22.0
CREME DE CACAO:		
(Bols)	1 fl. oz.	11.8
(Garnier)	1 fl. oz.	13.1
(Hiram Walker)	1 fl. oz.	15.0
(Leroux) white	1 fl. oz.	13.3
CREME DE CAFE (Leroux)	1 fl. oz.	13.6
CREME DE CASSIS:		
(Garnier)	1 fl. oz.	13.5
(Leroux)	1 fl. oz.	14.9
CREME DE MENTHE:		
(Bols)	1 fl. oz.	13.0
(Garnier)	1 fl. oz.	15.3
(Hiram Walker)	1 fl. oz.	11.2
(Leroux) green	1 fl. oz.	15.2
(Leroux) white	1 fl. oz.	12.8
CREPE, frozen (Mrs. Paul's):		
Clam	5½-oz. pkg.	21.6
Crab	5½-oz. pkg.	24.5

Food and Description	Measure or Quantity	Carbohydrates (grams)
Scallop	5½-oz. pkg.	25.2
Shrimp	5½-oz. pkg.	23.8
*CREPE MIX (Aunt Jemima)	6" crepe	15.0
CRISP RICE (Van Brode):		
Regular	1 oz.	24.9
Low sodium	1 oz.	25.7
CRISPY CRITTERS, cereal (Post)	1 cup	23.0
CRISPY RICE, cereal	1 cup	25.0
CROQUETTES, frozen, seafood (Mrs. Paul's)	½ of 6-oz. pkg.	23.9
CROUTON:		
(Arnold):		
American or Danish style	½ oz.	8.7
Bavarian or English style	½ oz.	9.5
French, Italian or Mexican style	½ oz.	9.5
Croutettes (Kellogg's)	.7 oz.	15.0
CUCUMBER:		
Eaten with skin	½ lb. cucumber	7.4
Pared, 10-oz. cucumber	7½" x 2" pared cucumber	6.6
Pared	3 slices	.8
CUMIN SEED (French's)	1 tsp.	.7
CUPCAKE:		
(Drake's) chocolate, cream-filled	1 cupcake	25.6
(Hostess):		
Chocolate	1 cupcake	29.9
Orange	1 cupcake	26.8
(Sara Lee) yellow, frozen	1 cupcake	27.9
(Tastykake):		
Chocolate	1 cupcake	33.0
Chocolate, chocolate creme-filled	1 cupcake	23.2
Coconut	1 cupcake	16.7
Creme-filled, chocolate buttercream	1 cupcake	23.1
Lemon creme-filled	1 cupcake	17.1
Vanilla creme-filled	1 cupcake	16.4
Vanilla Triplets	1 cupcake	16.1
*CUPCAKE MIX (Flako)	1 cupcake	25.0
CURAÇAO:		
(Bols)	1 fl. oz.	10.3
(Garnier)	1 fl. oz.	12.7
(Hiram Walker)	1 fl. oz.	11.8
CURRANT, dried, Zante (Del Monte)	½ cup	47.8
CURRANT JELLY (Smucker's)	1 T.	12.9
CUSTARD:		
Chilled, Swiss Miss, custard or egg flavor	4-oz. container	22.0
Chilled (Sealtest)	4-oz. serving	24.3
Frozen (See ICE CREAM)		
C. W. POST, cereal:		
Family-style	¼ cup	20.3
Family-style, with raisins	¼ cup	20.4

Food and Description	Measure or Quantity	Carbohydrates (grams)

D

Food and Description	Measure or Quantity	Carbohydrates (grams)
DAIQUIRI COCKTAIL:		
(Hiram Walker) 52½ proof	3 fl. oz.	12.0
(National Distillers) *Duet* 12½% alcohol	3 fl. oz.	18.0
(Party Tyme) 12½% alcohol	3 fl. oz.	7.3
Banana (Party Tyme) 12½% alcohol	3 fl. oz.	8.1
Dry mix (Bar-Tender's)	⅝-oz. serving	17.2
Dry mix (Holland House)	1 serving	17.0
Dry mix, banana:		
(Holland House)	1 serving	16.0
(Party Tyme)	1 serving	12.5
Liquid mix, canned:		
(Holland House)	2 fl. oz.	26.0
(Party Tyme)	2 fl. oz.	19.4
Liquid mix, canned, banana:		
(Holland House)	2 fl. oz.	36.0
(Party Tyme)	2 fl. oz.	14.6
*DANISH DESSERT (Junket)	½ cup	33.8
DATE:		
Whole (Cal-Date)	.8-oz. date	16.4
Imported Iraq (Bordo)	.2-oz. average date	46.0
Imported Iraq, dried (Bordo)	¼ cup	39.8
DE CHAUNAC WINE (Great Western) 12% alcohol	3 fl. oz.	2.4
DELAWARE WINE (Gold Seal) 12% alcohol	3 fl. oz.	2.6
DEVIL DOG (Drake's):		
Family	1 cake	24.9
Senior	1 cake	33.4
DILL SEED (French's)	1 tsp.	1.2
DING DONG (Hostess)	1 cake	21.1
DINNER, frozen (See individual listings such as **BEEF, CHINESE** or **ENCHILADA,** etc.)		
DIP:		
Bacon & horseradish:		
(Borden)	1 oz.	1.7
(Breakstone)	2 T.	1.3
(Kraft) *Teez*	1 oz.	1.6
Barbecue (Borden)	1 oz.	1.7
Blue cheese:		
(Breakstone)	2 T.	1.4
(Dean) Tang	1 oz.	2.3
(Kraft) *Teez*	1 oz.	1.3
Clam & lobster (Borden)	1 oz.	1.7
Cucumber & onion (Breakstone)	2 T.	1.7
Dill pickle (Kraft) *Ready Dip*	1 oz.	2.4

Food and Description	Measure or Quantity	Carbohydrates (grams)
Enchilada, *Fritos*	1 oz.	3.9
Garden spice (Borden)	1 oz.	2.1
Garlic (Dean)	1 oz.	2.0
Garlic (Kraft) *Teez*	1 oz.	1.5
Green goddess (Kraft) *Teez*	1 oz.	1.5
Jalapeño bean (Amigos)	3¼-oz. can	3.7
Jalapeño bean (Fritos)	1 oz.	3.7
Onion:		
(Borden) French	1 oz.	1.7
(Breakstone)	2 T.	1.9
(Dean) French	1 oz.	2.0
(Kraft) *Ready Dip*	1 oz.	2.0
(Sealtest) French	1 oz.	1.5
Pizza (Borden)	1 oz.	1.7
Skinny Dip (Dean)	1 oz.	2.4
Tasty tartar or Western Bar B-Q (Borden)	1 oz.	1.8
DIP MIX:		
Green onion (Lawry's)	1 pkg.	10.6
Guacamole (Lawry's)	1 pkg.	5.5
Toasted onion (Lawry's)	1 pkg.	9.8
DISTILLED LIQUOR, any brand:		
80 proof	1 fl. oz.	Tr.
86 proof	1 fl. oz.	Tr.
90 proof	1 fl. oz.	Tr.
94 proof	1 fl. oz.	Tr.
100 proof	1 fl. oz.	Tr.
DOUGHNUT:		
(Hostess):		
Cinnamon	1-oz. piece	14.5
Crunch	1-oz. piece	16.5
Plain	1-oz. piece	12.8
Powdered	1-oz. piece	15.1
Frozen (Morton):		
Bavarian cream	2-oz. piece	22.1
Boston creme	2.3-oz. piece	28.5
Chocolate iced	1½-oz. piece	19.6
Glazed	1½-oz. piece	19.2
Jelly	1.8-oz. piece	22.9
Mini	1.1-oz. piece	16.0
DOZY OATS:		
(Drake's)	1.1-oz. piece	22.4
(Drake's)	2-oz. piece	38.6
(Drake's)	2¼-oz. piece	44.2
DRAMBUIE (Hiram Walker)	1 fl. oz.	11.0
DREAMSICLE (Popsicle Industries)	2½ fl. oz.	13.1
DUMPLINGS, canned, dietetic:		
(Dia-Mel) stuffed with chicken	8-oz. can	28.0
(Featherweight) with chicken	8-oz. can	18.0

E

ECLAIR:		
Home recipe, with custard filling and chocolate icing	4 oz.	26.3
Frozen, chocolate (Rich's)	1 piece	30.0
EEL, smoked, meat only	4 oz.	0
EGG BEATERS (Fleischmann's)	¼ cup	3.0
EGG, CHICKEN:		
Raw, white only	1 large egg	.3
Raw, yolk only	1 large egg	.1
Boiled	1 large egg	.4
Fried in butter	1 large egg	.1
Omelet, mixed with milk & cooked in fat	1 large egg	1.5
Poached	1 large egg	.4
Scrambled, mixed with milk & cooked in fat	1 large egg	1.5
EGG FOO YONG (Chun King)	½ of 12-oz. pkg.	10.9
EGG MIX (Durkee):		
Omelet:		
*With bacon	½ of pkg.	10.0
*With cheese	½ of pkg.	24.0
*Puffy	½ of pkg.	11.0
Scrambled:		
Plain	.8-oz. pkg.	4.0
With bacon	1.3-oz. pkg.	6.0
EGG NOG, dairy:		
(Borden) 6% fat	½ cup	16.1
(Borden) 8% fat	½ cup	16.1
(Meadow Gold) 6% fat	½ cup	25.5
(Sealtest) 6% butterfat	½ cup	17.0
(Sealtest) 8% butterfat	½ cup	17.5
EGG-NOG ICE CREAM (Breyer's)	¼ pt.	16.0
EGGPLANT:		
Boiled	½ cup	4.1
Frozen:		
(Buitoni) parmigiana	4 oz.	16.2
(Mrs. Paul's) parmesan	½ of 11-oz. pkg.	21.5
(Mrs. Paul's) slices, breaded & fried	⅓ of 9-oz. pkg.	21.3
(Mrs. Paul's) sticks, breaded & fried	½ of 7-oz. pkg.	27.3
(Weight Watchers) parmigiana	13-oz. meal	25.1
EGG ROLL:		
(Chun King):		
Chicken	½-oz. roll	3.2
Meat & shrimp	½-oz. roll	3.7
Shrimp	½-oz. roll	3.8

Food and Description	Measure or Quantity	Carbohydrates (grams)
(La Choy):		
Chicken	.4-oz. roll	3.6
Lobster	.4-oz. roll	3.6
Meat & shrimp	.2-oz. roll	2.3
Meat & shrimp	.4-oz. roll	3.5
Shrimp	.4-oz. roll	3.7
Shrimp	2½-oz. roll	14.9
(Mow Sang):		
Chicken & mushroom	1 roll	7.0
Pork, barbecue	1 roll	6.0
EGG, SCRAMBLED, BREAKFAST		
(Swanson) with sausage & coffee cake	6¼-oz. breakfast	22.0
*EGGSTRA (Tillie Lewis)	1 large egg	4.0
ELDERBERRY, without stems	4 oz.	18.6
ELDERBERRY JELLY (Smucker's)	1 T.	13.3
ENCHILADA, frozen:		
Beef:		
(Banquet) with sauce	6-oz. bag	28.9
(Banquet) with cheese & chili gravy	2-lb. pkg.	118.2
Cheese:		
(Patio)	½ of 8-oz. pkg.	18.9
(Van de Kamp's) with sauce	7½-oz. pkg.	19.0
Chicken (Van de Kamp's) with sauce	7½-oz. pkg.	21.0
ENCHILADA DINNER:		
Beef:		
(Banquet)	12-oz. dinner	63.6
(Patio) 3-compartment	13-oz. dinner	34.0
(Swanson)	15-oz. dinner	72.0
(Van de Kamp's)	12-oz. dinner	41.0
Cheese:		
(Banquet)	12-oz. dinner	58.8
(Patio) 3-compartment	12-oz. dinner	40.0
(Van de Kamp's)	12-oz. dinner	38.0
ENCHILADA SAUCE MIX (Lawry's)	1 pkg.	27.3
ENDIVE, CURLY or ESCAROLE, cut up	½ cup	1.5
ESCAROLE SOUP, canned (Progresso), in chicken broth	8-oz. serving	1.0

F

FARINA:		
(Hi-O) dry, regular	¼ cup	33.4
Malt-O-Meal, dry, regular	1 oz.	21.1
Malt-O-Meal, dry, quick-cooking	1 oz.	22.0
(Pillsbury)	⅔ cup	26.0
FAT, cooking (Crisco; Fluffo)	1 T.	0

Food and Description	Measure or Quantity	Carbohydrates (grams)
FENNEL SEED (French's)	1 tsp.	1.3
FIG:		
Small	1½″ fig	7.7
Canned, regular pack (Del Monte) whole, solids & liq.	½ cup	28.1
Canned, dietetic (Featherweight) Kadota, water pack, solids & liq.	½ cup	15.0
Dried, chopped	½ cup	59.1
FIG JUICE, *RealFig*	½ cup	15.8
FIGURINES (Pillsbury) all flavors	1 bar	10.5
FILBERT, shelled	1 oz.	4.7
FISH AU GRATIN, frozen (Mrs. Paul's)	5-oz. serving	19.5
FISH CAKE (Mrs. Paul's):		
Breaded & fried	2-oz. cake	11.9
Thins, breaded & fried	½ of 10-oz. pkg.	35.3
FISH & CHIPS, frozen:		
(Gorton)	½ of 1-lb. pkg.	39.0
(Mrs. Paul's)	½ of 14-oz. pkg.	43.4
(Swanson)	10½-oz. dinner	40.0
(Swanson)	5-oz. pkg.	25.0
(Swanson) *Hungry Man*	15¾-oz. dinner	68.0
(Van de Kamp's) batter dipped, french fried	8-oz. serving	45.0
FISH CHOWDER, New England (Snow)	½ cup	8.6
FISH DINNER, frozen:		
(Banquet)	8¾-oz. dinner	43.6
(Morton)	9-oz. dinner	26.5
(Van de Kamp's) batter dipped, french fried	11-oz. dinner	39.0
FISH FILLET, frozen:		
(Mrs. Paul's):		
Batter fried	2¼-oz. piece	14.1
Breaded & fried	½ of 8-oz. pkg.	24.1
Buttered	2½-oz. piece	.9
Light batter, miniature	⅓ of 9-oz. pkg.	15.3
Parmesan	5-oz. piece	20.9
(Van de Kamp's):		
Batter dipped, french fried	3-oz. piece	12.5
Country seasoned	2.4-oz. piece	10.5
FISH FILLET DINNER (Van de Kamp's) batter dipped, french fried	12-oz. dinner	25.0
FISH KABOBS (Van de Kamp's):		
Batter dipped, french fried	.4-oz. piece	1.6
Country seasoned	.4-oz. piece	1.9
FISH STICK, frozen:		
(Commodore)	4 oz.	7.6
(Gorton)	½ of 8-oz. pkg.	8.0
(Mrs. Paul's) batter fried	1 stick	5.5
(Mrs. Paul's) breaded & fried	1 stick	4.1

Food and Description	*Measure or Quantity*	*Carbohydrates (grams)*
(Van de Kamp) batter dipped, french fried	1-oz. piece	3.2
FIT 'N FROSTY (Alba '77):		
Chocolate or strawberry	¾-oz. envelope	11.5
Vanilla	¾-oz. envelope	11.3
FLAN, chilled (Breakstone)	5-oz. container	37.5
FLOUNDER:		
Baked	4 oz.	0
(Mrs. Paul's) fillets, breaded & fried	2-oz. fillet	11.6
(Mrs. Paul's) with lemon butter	4¼-oz. serving	9.4
(Weight Watchers)	8½-oz. meal	13.0
(Weight Watchers)	16-oz. meal	14.1
FLOUR:		
(Aunt Jemima) self-rising	¼ cup	23.6
Ballard, self-rising	¼ cup	21.0
Bisquick (Betty Crocker)	¼ cup	19.0
Gold Medal (Betty Crocker) all-purpose	¼ cup	25.2
(Pillsbury) all-purpose	¼ cup	21.8
FRANKENBERRY, cereal	1 cup	24.0
FRANKFURTER:		
(Armour Star) all meat	1.6-oz. frankfurter	0
(Hormel):		
All beef	1.6-oz. frankfurter	.6
Wrangler	2-oz. frankfurter	.6
(Hygrade):		
Ball Park, beef	2-oz. frankfurter	6.1
All meat	1.6-oz. frankfurter	1.5
(Oscar Mayer):		
Beef	1.6-oz. frankfurter	1.4
Wiener	1.6-oz. frankfurter	1.3
Little Wiener	2" frankfurter	.3
(Swift)	1.6-oz. frankfurter	1.2
(Vienna) beef	1.5-oz. frankfurter	1.0
(Wilson)	1.6-oz. frankfurter	.8
(Wilson) skinless	1.6-oz. frankfurter	.8
Canned (Hormel)	⅙ of 12-oz. can	.4
FRANKS-N-BLANKETS (Durkee)	1 piece	1.0
FRENCH TOAST:		
(Aunt Jemima)	1.5-oz. slice	13.2
(Aunt Jemima) cinnamon swirl	1 slice	13.7
(Eggo)	1 slice	12.0
(Swanson) with sausage	4½-oz. breakfast	22.0
FROOT LOOPS, cereal (Kellogg's)	1 cup	25.0
FROSTED RICE, cereal (Kellogg's)	1 cup	26.0
FROSTI DEVILS (Drake's)	1 piece	22.0
FROSTY O's, cereal	1 oz.	24.0
FROZEN DESSERT:		
(*Charlotte Freeze*-Borden):		
Chocolate	⅓ pt.	23.1
Vanilla	⅓ pt.	21.0

Food and Description	Measure or Quantity	Carbohydrates (grams)
FRUIT BRUTE, cereal (General Mills)	1 cup	24.0
FRUIT COCKTAIL, canned, solids & liq.:		
Heavy syrup:		
(Del Monte)	½ cup	23.1
(Libby's)	½ cup	24.7
(Stokely-Van Camp)	½ cup	23.0
Dietetic pack:		
(Diet Delight) syrup pack	½ cup	14.3
(Diet Delight) water pack	½ cup	10.0
(Featherweight) juice pack	½ cup	12.0
(Libby's) water pack	½ cup	10.4
(S & W) *Nutradiet*, unsweetened	¼ cup	9.4
FRUIT CUP (Del Monte):		
Mixed fruits	5-oz. container	26.7
Peaches, diced	5-oz. container	27.8
FRUIT DOODLE (Drake's):		
Apple	1⅝-oz. pie	22.7
Cherry	1⅝-oz. pie	21.7
FRUIT, MIXED, frozen (Birds Eye)	5 oz.	34.5
FRUIT PUNCH:		
(Alegre)	8 fl. oz.	32.1
(Ann Page)	8 fl. oz.	30.4
(Lincoln) party	8 fl. oz.	34.8
FRUIT ROLL (La Choy)	.5-oz. roll	6.4
FRUIT SALAD:		
Bottled (Kraft)	4 oz.	13.3
(Del Monte):		
Fruits for salad	½ cup	23.0
Tropical	½ cup	26.0
(Libby's)	½ cup	24.0
Canned, dietetic pack:		
(Featherweight)	½ cup	13.0
(Diet Delight) unsweetened	½ cup	16.5
FUDGE ICE BAR: (Sealtest)	2½-fl.-oz. bar	19.0
FUDGSICLE (Popsicle Industries)	2½-fl.-oz. bar	23.6
FUNNY BONES (Drake's)	1¼-oz. cake	20.0
***FUNNY FACE**, all flavors	8 fl. oz.	20.0

G

GARLIC:		
Powder (French's)	1 tsp.	1.1
Spread (Lawry's)	1 T.	1.2
GAZPACHO SOUP (Crosse & Blackwell)	½ of 13-oz. can	1.0
GEFILTE FISH:		
(Manischewitz) 1-lb. jar	2.2-oz. piece	2.3
(Mother's) 1-lb. jar	2.7-oz. piece	2.3

Food and Description	Measure or Quantity	Carbohydrates (grams)
(Rokeach) liquid broth:		
27-oz. can	3⅓-oz. portion	.8
1-lb. or 1½-lb. can	4-oz. portion	.9
1½-lb. can	6-oz. portion	1.4
(Rokeach) *Old Vienna:*		
27-oz. can	3⅓-oz. portion	4.6
1-lb. or 1½-lb. can	4-oz. portion	5.5
1½-lb. can	6-oz. portion	8.2
GELATIN, dry (Ann Page)	1 envelope	0
GELATIN DESSERT:		
(Ann Page)	¼ of 3-oz. pkg.	19.0
*(Jells Best; Jell-O)	½ cup	18.0
*(Royal)	½ cup	18.9
Dietetic:		
(Dia-Mel) *Gel-a-Thin*	4-oz. container	.2
*(Dia-Mel) *Gel-a-Thin*	4-oz. serving	1.0
*(D-Zerta)	½ cup	0
(Estee)	½ cup	9.0
*(Louis Sherry) *Shimmer*	½ cup	1.0
GELATIN DRINK (Knox) orange	1 envelope	10.0
GERMAN DINNER (Swanson)	11¾-oz. dinner	40.0
GIMLET COCKTAIL:		
Canned (Party Tyme)		
17½% alcohol	2 fl. oz.	5.4
Dry mix (Holland House)	1 serving	17.0
Dry mix (Party Tyme)	½-oz. serving	11.5
GIN, SLOE:		
(Bols)	1 fl. oz.	4.7
(DeKuyper)	1 fl. oz.	5.2
(Hiram Walker)	1 fl. oz.	4.8
GIN & TONIC, canned (Party Tyme) 10% alcohol	2 fl. oz.	5.1
GINGER, powder (French's)	1 tsp.	1.2
GINGERBREAD MIX:		
(Betty Crocker)	⅑ of cake	36.0
(Dromedary)	2″ x 2″ square	19.0
(Pillsbury)	3″ square	36.0
GOLDEN GRAHAMS (General Mills)	1 cup	24.0
GOOD HUMOR:		
Chocolate eclair	3-oz. piece	25.0
Sandwich	2.5-oz. piece	34.0
Strawberry shortcake	3-oz. piece	21.0
Vanilla, chocolate coated	3-oz. piece	12.0
Whammy:		
Assorted	1.6-oz. piece	9.0
Chip crunch	1.6-oz. piece	10.0
Ice, assorted	1.5-oz. piece	13.0
GOOSE, roasted, meat & skin	4 oz.	0
GRAHAM CRAKOS, cereal	1 oz.	24.0
GRANOLA, cereal		
Heartland:		
Coconut	¼ cup	18.0

Food and Description	Measure or Quantity	Carbohydrates (grams)
Plain or raisin	¼ cup	18.0
Puffs, regular or cinnamon spice	½ cup	20.0
Nature Valley:		
Cinnamon & raisin	⅓ cup	19.0
Coconut & honey	⅓ cup	18.0
Fruit & nut	⅓ cup	20.0
Sun Country:		
With almonds	½ cup	34.0
With raisins	½ cup	37.0
Vita-Crunch:		
Regular	½ cup	45.1
Date	½ cup	47.0
Raisin	½ cup	46.4
GRANOLA BARS, *Nature Valley:*		
Cinnamon or honey 'n oats	.8-oz. bar	16.0
Coconut or peanut	.8-oz. bar	15.0
GRAPE:		
American type (slipskin)	3½" x 3" bunch	9.9
Canned, dietetic (Featherweight) water pack	½ cup	13.0
GRAPEADE, chilled (Sealtest)	8 fl. oz.	32.0
GRAPE DRINK:		
Canned:		
(Ann Page)	8 fl. oz.	31.1
(Hi-C)	6 fl. oz.	22.0
(Lincoln)	6 fl. oz.	26.2
(Wagner)	8 fl. oz.	32.4
*Mix (Hi-C)	6 fl. oz.	19.0
GRAPE JAM (Bama; Smucker's)	1 T.	13.5
GRAPE JELLY:		
Sweetened (Smucker's)	1 T.	13.3
Dietetic:		
(Dia-Mel)	1 tsp.	0
(Diet Delight)	1 T.	2.7
(Featherweight)	1 T.	4.0
(Featherweight) artificially sweetened	1 T.	1.0
(Louis Sherry) pure	1 tsp.	4.0
GRAPE JUICE, frozen:		
*(Minute Maid)	6 fl. oz.	25.0
*(Seneca)	½ cup	17.2
GRAPE-NUTS, cereal:		
Flakes	¾ cup	23.0
Nuggets	¾ cup	23.4
GRAPEFRUIT:		
Pink & red:		
Seeded type	½ med. grapefruit	11.9
Seedless type	½ med. grapefruit	12.8
White:		
Seeded type	½ med. grapefruit	11.7
Seedless type	½ med. grapefruit	11.9
Canned, syrup pack (Del Monte)	½ cup	17.5

Food and Description	Measure or Quantity	Carbohydrates (grams)
Canned, unsweetened:		
(Del Monte; Diet Delight) sections	½ cup	11.0
(Featherweight) sections	½ cup	9.0
(Tillie Lewis)	½ cup	11.2
GRAPEFRUIT DRINK, canned:		
(Ann Page) natural	6 fl. oz.	20.7
(Lincoln)	6 fl. oz.	26.1
GRAPEFRUIT JUICE:		
Fresh, pink, red or white	½ cup	11.3
Bottled, sweetened (Kraft)	½ cup	14.0
Canned, sweetened:		
(Del Monte)	6 fl. oz.	20.8
(Stokely-Van Camp)	½ cup	16.2
Canned, unsweetened:		
(Del Monte; Ocean Spray)	6 fl. oz.	16.6
(Featherweight)	½ cup	9.0
*Frozen, unsweetened (Minute Maid)	6 fl. oz.	18.3
GRASSHOPPER COCKTAIL MIX		
(Holland House)	1 serving	17.0
GRAVES WINE (B&G; Cruse)	3 fl. oz.	.6
GRAVY:		
Beef:		
(Ann Page)	10½-oz. can	18.3
(Franco-American)	10¼-oz. can	15.4
Brown:		
(Dawn Fresh) with mushroom broth	2 oz.	4.0
(Franco-American) with onion	10½-oz. can	21.0
(La Choy)	5-oz. can	101.3
Ready Gravy	¼ cup	7.4
Chicken:		
(Franco-American)	10½-oz. can	15.8
Giblet (Franco-American)	10½-oz. can	15.8
Mushroom (Franco-American)	10½-oz. can	21.0
GRAVYMASTER	1 fl. oz.	14.2
GRAVY with MEAT or TURKEY:		
Canned:		
(Bunker Hill):		
Beef chunks	15-oz. can	16.0
Chopped beef	10½-oz. can	10.0
Sliced beef	15-oz. can	16.0
(Morton House):		
Sliced beef	½ of 12½-oz. can	8.0
Sliced pork	½ of 12½-oz. can	9.0
Sliced turkey	½ of 12½-oz. can	7.0
Frozen:		
(Banquet):		
Giblet gravey & sliced turkey	5-oz. bag	5.3
Sliced beef	2-lb. pkg.	34.5

Food and Description	Measure or Quantity	Carbohydrates (grams)
(Green Giant):		
Sliced beef, *Toast Topper*	5-oz. serving	5.7
Sliced turkey, *Toast Topper*	5-oz. serving	6.7
GRAVY MIX:		
Au jus:		
(Ann Page)	¾-oz. pkg.	10.9
(Durkee)	1 pkg.	13.0
(Durkee) *Roastin' Bag*	1-oz. pkg.	14.0
(French's) *Gravy Makins*	¾-oz. pkg.	12.0
Brown:		
(Ann Page)	¾-oz. pkg.	12.0
(Durkee)	.8-oz. pkg.	10.0
(Durkee) with mushrooms	.7-oz. pkg.	11.0
(Durkee) with onions	18-oz. pkg.	13.0
*(Ehler's)	¼ cup	3.5
(French's) *Gravy Makins*	¾-oz. pkg.	13.7
*(Spatini)	1-oz. cup	3.0
Chicken:		
(Ann Page)	1-oz. pkg.	16.7
(Durkee)	1 pkg.	14.0
*(Pillsbury)	¼ cup	3.0
*Home-style (Pillsbury)	¼ cup	3.0
Mushroom (Durkee)	1 pkg.	11.0
Onion (Durkee)	1 pkg.	15.0
Pork (Durkee)	1-oz. pkg.	14.0
Pot roast (Durkee) *Roastin' Bag*	1.5-oz. pkg.	25.0
Swiss steak (Durkee)	1-oz. pkg.	16.0
Turkey (Durkee)	1-oz. pkg.	14.0
GRENADINE (Garnier) no alcohol	1 fl. oz.	26.0
GUAVA	1 guava	11.7

H

HADDOCK:		
Fried, breaded	4″ x 3″ x ½″ fillet	5.8
Frozen:		
(Banquet)	8¾-oz. dinner	45.4
(Mrs. Paul's) breaded & fried	2-oz. fillet	11.8
(Mrs. Paul's) buttered fillets	½ of 10-oz. pkg.	1.2
(Van de Kamp's) batter		
dipped, french fried	2.4-oz. piece	8.0
(Weight Watchers)	16-oz. meal	13.2
Smoked	4 oz.	0
HALIBUT:		
Broiled	4″ x 3″ x ½″ steak	0
Frozen (Van de Kamp's) batter		
dipped, french fried	1.3-oz. piece	5.7
HAM:		
Boiled:		
(Hormel)	1 oz.	0
Chopped, sliced (Hormel)	1 oz.	<1.0

Food and Description	Measure or Quantity	Carbohydrates (grams)
Canned:		
(Armour Golden Star)	1 oz.	0
(Armour Star)	1 oz.	0
(Hormel) *Tender Chunk*	1 oz.	0
(Oscar Mayer) *Jubilee*, extra lean, cooked	4-oz. slice	.5
(Swift) *Hostess*	3½-oz. slice	.8
(Swift) *Premium*	1¾-oz. slice	.3
Deviled:		
(Armour Star)	1 oz.	0
(Libby's)	1 oz.	.3
(Underwood)	¼ of 4½-oz. can	Tr.
Packaged, chopped (Oscar Mayer)	1-oz. slice	.3
Packaged (Oscar Mayer) *Jubilee*, boneless	½-lb slice	0
HAM & CHEESE (Oscar Mayer):		
Loaf	1-oz. slice	.3
Spread	1 oz.	.7
HAM DINNER:		
(Banquet)	10-oz. dinner	47.7
(Morton)	10-oz. dinner	56.9
(Swanson)	10¼-oz. dinner	47.0
HAMBURGER (See McDONALD'S and BURGER KING)		
HAMBURGER MIX:		
(Ann Page):		
Beef noodle	⅕ of 7-oz. pkg.	48.2
Chili tomato	⅕ of 8-oz. pkg.	32.5
Potato stroganoff	⅕ of 7-oz. pkg.	28.2
Hamburger Helper (General Mills):		
Beef noodle	⅕ of pkg.	26.0
Chili tomato	⅕ of pkg.	29.0
Hamburger stew	⅕ of pkg.	23.0
Lasagne	⅕ of pkg.	32.0
Rice oriental	⅕ of pkg.	35.0
Make A Better Burger (Lipton) mildly seasoned or onion	1 patty	3.0
HAMBURGER SEASONING MIX:		
(Durkee)	1-oz. pkg.	15.0
*(Durkee)	1 cup	7.5
(French's)	1-oz. pkg.	20.0
HAM SALAD, canned (Carnation)	1½ oz.	3.4
HAM SALAD SPREAD (Oscar Mayer)	1 oz.	3.0
HAWAIIAN PUNCH:		
Canned:		
Cherry	6 fl. oz.	22.9
Grape	6 fl. oz.	23.4
Orange	6 fl. oz.	24.4
Red	6 fl. oz.	21.3

Food and Description	Measure or Quantity	Carbohydrates (grams)
Very berry	6 fl. oz.	21.6
*Mix, red punch	8 fl. oz.	25.0
HEADCHEESE (Oscar Mayer)	1 oz.	.6
HEARTLAND, cereal (See GRANOLA)		
HERRING, canned (Vita):		
Bismarck, drained	5-oz. jar	6.9
Cocktail, drained	8-oz. jar	24.8
In cream sauce	8-oz. jar	18.1
In wine sauce, drained	8-oz. jar	16.6
Lunch, drained	8-oz. jar	13.1
Matjes, drained	8-oz. jar	26.2
Party snacks, drained	8-oz. jar	16.6
Tastee Bits, drained	8-oz. jar	24.7
HERRING, smoked, kippered	4 oz.	0
HICKORY NUT, shelled	1 oz.	3.6
HOB NOB, any flavor (Drake's)	1 piece	9.1
HO-HO (Hostess)	1-oz cake	16.5
HOMINY GRITS:		
Dry:		
(Albers)	1½ oz.	33.0
(Aunt Jemima/Quaker)	3 T.	22.4
Quaker instant	.8-oz. packet	17.7
(Quaker) instant, with imitation bacon or ham	1-oz. packet	21.6
Cooked	1 cup	27.0
HONEY, strained	1 T.	16.5
HONEYCOMB, cereal	1⅛ cups	25.1
HONEYDEW	2" x 7" wedge	7.2
HOPPING JOHN (Green Giant)	⅓ cup	16.7
HORSERADISH:		
Regular (Kraft)	1 oz.	.4
Cream-style (Kraft)	1 oz.	.7
*HOT DOG BEAN SOUP (Campbell)	8-oz. serving	20.0
HUSH PUPPY, refrigerated (Borden)	1 piece	10.7

I

ICE CREAM & FROZEN CUSTARD: (See also listing by flavor or brand name or FROZEN DESSERT)		
(Dean) 10.4% fat	1 cup	41.1
ICE CREAM BAR, chocolate-coated (Sealtest)	2½-fl.-oz. bar	12.0
ICE CREAM CONE, cone only:		
(Comet)	1 piece	3.9
Rolled sugar (Comet)	1 piece	10.2
ICE CREAM CUP, cup only (Comet)	1 piece	4.1
ICE CREAM SANDWICH (Sealtest)	3 fl. oz.	26.0

Food and Description	Measure or Quantity	Carbohydrates (grams)
ICE MILK:		
Hardened	¼ pt.	14.6
Soft-serve	¼ pt.	19.6
(Borden):		
2.5% fat, any flavor	¼ pt.	7.6
3.25% fat, any flavor	¼ pt.	18.1
Lite Line	¼ pt.	16.0
(Dean):		
Count Calorie	¼ pt.	8.6
5% fat	¼ pt.	17.5
Light 'n Easy:		
Chocolate	½ cup	17.7
Strawberry	½ cup	17.7
Vanilla	½ cup	17.2
(Meadow Gold) vanilla, 4% fat	¼ pt.	16.5
(Sealtest) *Light 'n Lively:*		
Banana	¼ pt.	19.7
Banana strawberry twirl, chocolate, toffee, vanilla fudge royale	¼ pt.	20.0
Buttered almond, caramel nut	¼ pt.	18.0
Cherry pineapple, coffee, orange-pineapple, peach, strawberry, vanilla, vanilla with chocolate and strawberry	¼ pt.	18.0
ICE MILK BAR, chocolate-coated (Sealtest)	2½-fl.-oz. bar	14.0
ICE STICK, Twin Pops (Sealtest)	3 fl. oz.	18.0
INTERNATIONAL DESSERTS (Sara Lee):		
Chocolate Bavarian	⅛ of pkg.	22.6
French cream cheese	⅛ of pkg.	24.9
Lemon Bavarian	⅛ of pkg.	22.3
Strawberry French cream cheese	⅛ of pkg.	27.5
ITALIAN DINNER:		
(Banquet)	11-oz. dinner	44.6
(Swanson)	13-oz. dinner	55.0

J

JAM, sweetened (Ann Page) all flavors	1 tsp.	4.8
JELLY, sweetened:		
(Ann Page) all flavors	1 T.	4.5
(Crosse & Blackwell) all flavors	1 T.	12.8
(Smucker's) all flavors	1 T.	12.4
JERUSALEM ARTICHOKE, pared	4 oz.	18.9
JOHANNESBERG REISLING:		
(Deinhard)	3 fl. oz.	4.5
(Inglenook)	3 fl. oz.	.9

Food and Description	Measure or Quantity	Carbohydrates (grams)
JUNIORS (Tastykake):		
Chocolate	2¾-oz. pkg.	70.8
Coconut	2¾-oz. pkg.	83.5
Koffee kake	2½-oz. pkg.	59.7
Lemon	2¾-oz. pkg.	84.8

K

KABOOM, cereal (General Mills)	1 cup	24.0
KALE:		
Boiled, leaves only	4 oz.	6.9
Chopped (Birds Eye) frozen	⅓ pkg.	5.0
KARO syrup:		
Dark corn	1 T.	15.0
Dark corn	½ cup	121.5
Imitation maple	1 T.	14.6
Imitation maple	½ cup	117.7
Light corn	1 T.	14.9
Light corn	½ cup	125.0
Pancake & waffle syrup	1 T.	14.9
Pancake & waffle syrup	½ cup	120.6
KEFIR (Alta-Dena Dairy):		
Plain	1 cup	13.0
Flavored	1 cup	24.0
KIDNEY:		
Beef, braised	4 oz.	.9
Calf, raw	4 oz.	.1
Lamb, raw	4 oz.	1.0
KIELBASA (Vienna)	2½ oz.	1.1
KING VITAMAN, cereal	¾ cup	23.3
KIRSCH, liqueur (Garnier)	1 fl. oz.	8.8
KIX, cereal	1½ cups	24.0
KNOCKWURST	1 oz.	.6
*KOOL-AID (General Foods):		
Unsweetened	8 fl. oz.	25.0
Sweetened, all flavors but tropical punch	8 fl. oz.	23.2
Sweetened, tropical punch	8 fl. oz.	24.5
KUMQUAT, flesh & skin	5 oz.	19.4

L

LAKE COUNTRY, wine (Taylor):		
Gold, 12% alcohol	3 fl. oz.	5.4
Pink, 12.5% alcohol	3 fl. oz.	4.8
Red, 12.5% alcohol	3 fl. oz.	4.8
White, 12.5% alcohol	3 fl. oz.	4.2
LAMB	Any quantity	0
LAMB STEW, canned, dietetic (Featherweight)	7¼-oz. can	23.0

Food and Description	Measure or Quantity	Carbohydrates (grams)
LARD	1 T.	0
LASAGNE:		
Canned (Nalley's)	8-oz. can	27.2
Frozen:		
(Buitoni)	8-oz. serving	38.9
(Green Giant) with meat sauce, *Bake 'n Serve*	7-oz. serving	27.8
(Green Giant) with meat sauce, boil-in-bag	9-oz. entree	32.2
(Ronzoni)	⅛ of 26-oz. pkg.	22.0
(Swanson) with meat, *Hungry Man*	17¾-oz. dinner	86.0
(Swanson) *Hungry Man*	12¾-oz. entree	51.0
(Weight Watchers)	13-oz. meal	35.1
Seasoning mix (Lawry's)	1.1-oz. pkg.	19.6
LAZY BONE (Drake's)	.9-oz. cake	15.2
LEEKS	4 oz.	12.7
LEMON:		
Whole	2⅛" lemon	11.7
Peeled	2⅛" lemon	6.1
LEMONADE:		
Canned, *Country Time*	6 fl. oz.	16.7
Frozen:		
*Country Time, regular & pink	6 fl. oz.	17.0
*Minute Maid	6 fl. oz.	19.6
*(Seneca)	6 fl. oz.	19.5
*Mix:		
Country Time, regular & pink	6 fl. oz.	16.5
(Hi-C)	6 fl. oz.	19.0
Kool-Aid, sweetened, regular or pink	6 fl. oz.	18.8
Kool-Aid, unsweetened, regular or pink	6 fl. oz.	16.7
Lemon Tree (Lipton)	6 fl. oz.	16.5
LEMON EXTRACT (Virginia Dare)	1 tsp.	0
LEMON JUICE:		
(Sunkist)	1 lemon	4.0
ReaLemon	1 T.	.8
LEMON-LIME DRINK:		
(Wagner)	6 fl. oz.	21.6
Mix (Wyler's)	3-oz. pouch	84.6
LEMON PEEL, candied	1 oz.	22.9
LENTIL SOUP:		
(Crosse & Blackwell) with ham	½ of 13-oz. can	13.0
*(Manischewitz)	1 cup	29.3
(Progresso)	1 cup	22.0
LETTUCE:		
Bibb or Boston	4" head	4.1
Cos or Romaine, shredded or broken into pieces	½ cup	.8
Grand Rapids, Salad Bowl or Simpson	2 large leaves	1.8

Food and Description	Measure or Quantity	Carbohydrates (grams)
Iceberg, New York or Great Lakes	¼ of 4¾" head	3.3
LIEBFRAUMILCH WINE:		
(Anheuser)	3 fl. oz.	.9
(Deinhard)	3 fl. oz.	3.6
(Julius Kayser) Glockenspiel	3 fl. oz.	1.8
LIFE, cereal (Quaker)	⅔ cup	19.7
LIME, peeled	2" dia	4.9
*LIMEADE (Minute Maid)	6 fl. oz.	20.1
LIME ICE, home recipe	4 oz.	37.0
LIME JUICE, *ReaLime*	1 T.	.5
LINGUINI IN CLAM SAUCE (Ronzoni)	4-oz. serving	16.0
LIVER:		
Beef, fried	6½" x 2⅜" x ⅜" slice	4.5
Beef, cooked (Swift)	3.2-oz. serving	3.1
Calf, fried	6½" x 2⅜" x ⅜" slice	3.4
Chicken, simmered	2" x 2" x ⅝" liver	.8
LIVERWURST SPREAD (Underwood)	1 oz.	1.1
LOBSTER:		
Cooked, meat only	1 cup	.4
Canned, meat only	4 oz.	.3
Frozen, South African Lobster tail:		
3 in 8-oz. pkg.	1 piece	.2
4 in 8-oz. pkg.	1 piece	.1
5 in 8-oz. pkg.	1 piece	<.1
LOBSTER NEWBURG	1 cup	12.8
LOBSTER PASTE, canned	1 oz.	.4
LOBSTER SALAD	4 oz.	2.6
LOBSTER SOUP, cream of (Crosse & Blackwell)	½ of 13-oz. can	6.5
LOG CABIN, syrup:		
Regular	1 T.	13.1
Buttered	1 T.	13.0
Maple-honey	1 T.	13.9
LOQUAT, fresh, flesh only	2 oz.	17.0
LOVE BIRD COCKTAIL MIX (Holland House)	1 serving	17.0
LUCKY CHARMS, cereal (General Mills)	1 cup	24.0
LUNCHEON MEAT (See also individual listings, e.g., **BOLOGNA**):		
All meat (Oscar Mayer)	1-oz. slice	.7
Bar-B-Que loaf (Oscar Mayer)	1-oz. slice	1.7
Ham & cheese (See **HAM & CHEESE**)		
Honey loaf (Oscar Mayer)	1-oz. slice	1.1
Liver cheese (Oscar Mayer)	1.3-oz. slice	.5
Meat loaf	1 oz.	.9
New England brand sliced sausage	.8-oz. slice	.3

Food and Description	Measure or Quantity	Carbohydrates (grams)
Old fashioned loaf (Oscar Mayer)	1-oz. slice	2.3
Olive loaf (Oscar Mayer)	1-oz. slice	2.6
Peppered beef (Vienna)	1 oz.	.4
Pickle & pimiento:		
(Hormel)	1 oz.	.3
(Oscar Mayer)	1-oz. slice	2.9
Spiced (Hormel)	1 oz.	<1.0

M

MACADAMIA NUT (Royal Hawaiian)	1 oz.	4.6
MACARONI, cooked:		
8-10 minutes, firm	1 cup	39.1
14-20 minutes, tender	1 cup	32.3
MACARONI & BEEF:		
Canned, in tomato sauce:		
(Bounty)	7¾-oz. can	29.7
(Franco-American) *Beefy Mac*	7½-oz. can	28.0
Frozen:		
(Banquet)	12-oz. dinner	55.1
(Banquet) buffet	2-lb. pkg.	106.4
(Green Giant)	9-oz. entree	30.7
(Swanson)	12-oz. dinner	55.0
MACARONI & CHEESE:		
Canned:		
(Franco-American)	7⅜-oz. serving	24.0
(Franco-American) elbow	7⅜-oz. serving	23.8
Frozen:		
(Banquet) buffet	2-lb. pkg.	110.9
(Banquet) dinner	12-oz. dinner	45.6
(Green Giant) bag	9-oz. entree	35.8
(Green Giant) oven bake	6-oz. serving	23.7
(Morton)	8-oz. casserole	34.1
(Swanson)	12½-oz. dinner	55.0
(Van De Kamp's)	10-oz. pkg.	46.0
Mix:		
(Ann Page) dinner	¼ of 7¼-oz. pkg.	37.5
(Betty Crocker)	¼ pkg.	37.0
*(Betty Crocker)	¼ pkg.	38.0
(Golden Grain) deluxe	¼ of 7¼-oz. pkg.	38.1
*(Pennsylvania Dutch Brand)	½ cup	25.0
*(Prince)	¾ cup	34.6
MACARONI DINNER, frozen:		
(Morton) & beef	10-oz. dinner	45.5
(Morton) & cheese	11-oz. dinner	53.1
(Weight Watchers) ziti	13-oz. meal	39.1
MACARONI SALAD, canned (Nalley's)	4 oz.	13.9
MACKEREL, Atlantic, broiled with fat	8½" x 2½" x ½" fillet	0

Food and Description	Measure or Quantity	Carbohydrates (grams)
MADEIRA WINE (Leacock)	3 fl. oz.	6.3
MAI TAI COCKTAIL:		
Canned:		
(Lemon Hart) 48 proof	3 fl. oz.	15.6
(National Distillers-*Duet*)		
12½% alcohol	8-fl.-oz. can	28.8
Dry mix:		
(Bar-Tender's; Holland House)	1 serving	17.0
(Party Tyme)	½-oz. serving	11.8
Liquid mix, canned		
(Holland House)	1½ fl. oz.	12.0
MALTED MILK MIX:		
Chocolate (Carnation)	3 heaping tsps.	18.0
Natural (Carnation)	3 heaping tsps.	15.6
MALT LIQUOR:		
Champale, regular	12 fl. oz.	12.2
Schlitz	12 fl. oz.	13.7
MANDARIN ORANGE		
(See TANGERINE)		
MANGO, fresh	1 med. mango	22.5
MANHATTAN COCKTAIL:		
Canned:		
(Hiram Walker) 55 proof	3 fl. oz.	3.0
(National Distillers-*Duet*)		
20% alcohol	8-fl.-oz. can	11.2
(Party Tyme) 20% alcohol	2 fl. oz.	1.5
Brandy (National Distillers-*Duet*) 20% alcohol	8-fl.-oz. can	8.0
Dry mix (Bar-Tender's)	1 serving	5.6
Liquid mix, canned		
(Holland House)	1½ fl. oz.	10.5
MAPLE SYRUP (Cary's)	1 T.	15.7
MARGARINE:		
Regular	1 oz.	.1
Regular	1 T.	<.1
Regular	1 pat (1″ x 1.3″ x 1″, 5 grams)	Tr.
MARGARINE, IMITATION:		
(Fleischmann's; Mazola, Weight Watchers)	1 T.	0
(Parkay)	1 T.	0
MARGARINE, WHIPPED		
(Blue Bonnet; Miracle; Parkay)	1 T.	0
MARGARITA COCKTAIL:		
Canned:		
(National Distillers-*Duet*)		
12½% alcohol	8-fl.-oz. can	20.0
(Party Tyme) 12½% alcohol	2 fl. oz.	5.7
Dry Mix:		
(Bar-Tender's; Holland House)	1 serving	17.3
(Party Tyme)	½-oz. serving	11.5

Food and Description	Measure or Quantity	Carbohydrates (grams)
Liquid Mix:		
(Holland House)	1½ fl. oz.	14.2
(Party Tyme)	2 fl. oz.	14.9
MARINADE MIX:		
(Adolph's) chicken	1-oz. packet	14.4
(Adolph's) meat	.8-oz. pkg.	8.5
(Durkee) meat	1-oz. pkg.	9.0
(French's) meat	1-oz. pkg.	16.0
(Lawry's) beef	1.6-oz. pkg.	15.1
MARJORAM (French's)	1 tsp.	.8
MARMALADE:		
Sweetened:		
(Ann Page)	1 T.	14.8
(Bama; Smucker's)	1 T.	13.5
(Keiller)	1 T.	15.0
Dietetic:		
(Dia-Mel)	1 T.	0
(Louis Sherry)	1 tsp.	0
(Tillie Lewis)	1 T.	3.0
MARSHMALLOW FLUFF	1 heaping tsp.	15.6
MARTINI COCKTAIL:		
Gin:		
(Hiram Walker) 67.5 proof	3 fl. oz.	.6
(National Distillers-*Duet*)		
21% alcohol	8-fl.-oz. can	1.6
(Party Tyme) 24% alcohol	3 fl. oz.	0
Liquid mix (Holland House)	2 fl. oz.	5.1
Liquid mix (Party Tyme)	2 fl. oz.	3.2
Vodka:		
(Hiram Walker) 60 proof	3 fl. oz.	0
(National Distillers-*Duet*)		
20% alcohol	8-fl.-oz. can	1.6
(Party Tyme) 21% alcohol	3 fl. oz.	0
MAYONNAISE:		
(Ann Page; Dia-Mel; Sultana)	1 T.	.1
(Best Foods *Real*;		
Hellmann's *Real*)	1 T.	<.1
(Weight Watchers) imitation	1 T.	1.0
MAYPO, cereal:		
30-second	¼ cup	16.4
Vermont-style	¼ cup	22.0
McDONALD'S:		
Big Mac	1 hamburger	39.0
Cheeseburger	1 cheeseburger	30.8
Cookies, *McDonaldland*	1 package	45.4
Egg McMuffin	1 serving	26.0
English muffin, buttered	1 muffin	28.3
Filet-O-Fish	1 sandwich	34.3
French fries	1 regular-serving	25.8
Hamburger	1 hamburger	30.2
Hot cakes with butter & syrup	1 serving	89.0

Food and Description	Measure or Quantity	Carbohydrates (grams)
Pie:		
Apple	1 pie	31.1
Cherry	1 pie	32.5
Quarter Pounder	1 hamburger	33.0
Quarter Pounder, with cheese	1 hamburger	33.1
Sausage, pork	1 serving	.5
Scrambled eggs	1 serving	1.9
Shake:		
Chocolate	1 serving	59.8
Strawberry	1 serving	57.3
Vanilla	1 serving	51.7
MEATBALL DINNER OR ENTREE:		
(Swanson)	11¾-oz. dinner	35.0
(Swanson)	9½-oz. entree	26.0
MEATBALL SEASONING MIX:		
(Durkee):		
*Italian	¼ of pkg.	2.3
*Italian, with cheese	¼ of pkg.	2.3
(French's)	1½-oz. pkg.	28.0
MEATBALL STEW, canned:		
(Libby's)	⅓ of 24-oz. can	24.5
(Morton House)	⅓ of 24-oz. can	18.0
MEAT LOAF DINNER:		
(Banquet)	11-oz. dinner	29.0
(Banquet) *Man-Pleaser*	19-oz. dinner	63.6
(Morton)	11-oz. dinner	28.1
(Morton) *Country Table*	15-oz. dinner	59.7
(Swanson)	10¾-oz. dinner	48.0
MEAT LOAF SEASONING MIX:		
(Contadina)	3¾-oz. pkg.	72.8
(French's)	1½-oz. pkg.	40.0
MEAT POTTED:		
(Armour Star)	3-oz. can	0
(Libby's)	1 oz.	.3
MEAT TENDERIZER:		
(Adolph's)	1 tsp.	.5
(French's)	1 tsp.	<.5
MELBA TOAST, salted:		
Garlic, onion or plain (Keebler)	1 piece	1.5
Garlic, onion or white rounds (Old London)	1 piece	1.8
Pumpernickel, rye, wheat or white (Old London)	1 piece	3.4
Sesame (Keebler)	1 piece	1.4
Sesame, flat (Old London)	1 piece	3.0
Sesame, round (Old London)	1 piece	1.6
MELON BALL, in syrup, frozen	½ cup	18.2
MEXICAN DINNER, frozen:		
(Banquet)	16-oz. dinner	73.5
(Banquet) combination	12-oz. dinner	72.1
(Swanson) combination	16-oz. dinner	72.0

Food and Description	Measure or Quantity	Carbohydrates (grams)
(Van de Kamp's)	12-oz. dinner	47.0
(Van de Kamp's) combination	11-oz. dinner	37.0
MILK, CONDENSED, *Dime Brand, Eagle Brand; Magnolia Brand*	1 T.	9.5
MILK, DRY, nonfat instant:		
*(Alba; Carnation; Pet)	1 cup	12.0
Low sodium (Featherweight)	⅔ oz.	10.0
MILK, EVAPORATED (Carnation):		
Regular	1 fl. oz.	3.0
Low fat	1 fl. oz.	3.0
Skim	1 fl. oz.	3.5
MILK, FRESH:		
(Dean; Sealtest) whole, 3.5% fat	1 cup	11.0
(Sealtest) extra rich vitamin D	1 cup	11.0
Skim:		
(Borden)	1 cup	13.6
(Borden) *Pro-Line*, 2% fat	1 cup	14.2
(Dean) .5% fat	1 cup	11.7
(Dean) 2% fat	1 cup	12.5
(Meadow Gold) vitamins A & D	1 cup	11.0
(Meadow Gold) *Viva*, 2% fat, vitamins A & D	1 cup	12.0
(Sealtest)	1 cup	11.3
(Sealtest) protein fortified, vitamins A & D	1 cup	10.0
Buttermilk:		
(Borden) 1.0% fat	1 cup	12.4
(Dean)	1 cup	11.5
(Sealtest)	1 cup	11.0
Light 'n Lively, protein fortified	1 cup	14.0
(Sealtest) protein fortified	1 cup	12.0
Chocolate milk:		
(Dean) with whole milk	1 cup	25.5
(Dean) with skim milk, 1% fat	1 cup	27.9
(Sealtest) with skim milk, .5% fat	1 cup	26.2
(Sealtest) vitamin D	1 cup	22.0
MINESTRONE SOUP:		
*(Ann Page)	1 cup	12.8
(Campbell) *Chunky*	19-oz. can	50.0
*(Campbell) condensed	8-oz. serving	12.0
(Crosse & Blackwell)	6½-oz. serving	18.0
MINI-WHEATS, cereal:		
Frosted	4 biscuits	24.0
Toasted	5 biscuits	22.0
MINT LEAVES	½ oz.	.8
MOLASSES (Brer Rabbit) dark	1 T.	10.6
MORTADELLA, sausage	1 oz.	.2
MOSELLE WINE (Great Western)	3 fl. oz.	2.9
MOST, cereal	1 oz.	22.0
MUFFIN:		
Blueberry (Morton) frozen	1.6-oz. muffin	22.9

Food and Description	Measure or Quantity	Carbohydrates (grams)
Blueberry (Morton) frozen, rounds	1.5-oz. muffin	20.9
Bran (Arnold) *Orowheat*	2.3-oz. muffin	30.0
Corn:		
(Morton) frozen	1.7-oz. muffin	20.3
(Morton) frozen, rounds	1.5-oz. muffin	20.9
(Thomas')	2-oz. muffin	25.8
English:		
(Arnold)	2-oz. muffin	25.0
(Pepperidge Farm)	1 muffin	27.0
(Thomas')	2-oz. muffin	26.6
(Thomas') onion	2-oz. muffin	26.3
Honey butter (Arnold)	2.2-oz. muffin	30.0
Plain	1.4-oz. muffin	16.9
Raisin (Arnold)	2.5-oz. muffin	30.0
Raisin (Wonder) rounds	2-oz. muffin	28.0
Sourdough (Wonder)	2-oz. muffin	27.0
MUFFIN MIX:		
Blueberry:		
*(Betty Crocker) wild	½ pkg.	19.0
(Duncan Hines)	½₂ pkg.	4.0
*Cinnamon nut (Betty Crocker)	½₂ pkg.	21.0
Corn:		
*(Betty Crocker)	½₂ pkg.	25.0
*(Dromedary)	1 muffin	20.0
*(Flako)	1 muffin	23.0
*Sunkist orange (Betty Crocker)	½₂ pkg.	26.0
MUG-O-LUNCH (General Mills):		
Macaroni & cheese sauce	1 pouch	40.0
Noodles & beef flavored sauce	1 pouch	29.0
Spaghetti & tomato sauce	1 pouch	29.0
MUSCATEL WINE (Gallo)		
14% alcohol	3 fl. oz.	7.9
MUSHROOM:		
Raw, whole	½ lb.	9.7
Raw, trimmed, slices	½ cup	1.5
Canned:		
(Green Giant)	2-oz. serving	1.7
(Shady Oaks)	4-oz. can	2.0
Frozen (Green Giant) whole,		
in butter sauce	½ of 6-oz. pkg.	2.6
MUSHROOM, CHINESE, dried	1 oz.	18.9
MUSHROOM SOUP:		
*(Ann Page) cream of	1 cup	10.2
*(Campbell) cream of	8-oz. serving	8.8
(Campbell) cream of, *Soup*		
For One	7½-oz. can	12.0
*(Campbell) golden	8-oz. serving	8.8
(Crosse & Blackwell) cream		
of bisque	½ of 13-oz. can	8.0
*(Manischewitz) barley	8-oz. serving	12.2

Food and Description	Measure or Quantity	Carbohydrates (grams)
Dietetic:		
(Campbell) cream of, low sodium	7½-oz. can	10.0
*(Dia-Mel)	8-oz. serving	9.0
(Featherweight)	8-oz. can	18.0
MUSHROOM SOUP MIX:		
*(Lipton) beef	8-oz.	7.0
*(Lipton) cream of, Cup-a-Soup	6 fl. oz.	11.0
*(Nestlé's) Souptime	6 fl. oz.	9.0
MUSSEL, in shell	1 lb.	7.2
MUSTARD:		
Powder (French's)	1 tsp.	.3
Prepared:		
Brown (French's; Gulden's; Grey Poupon)	1 tsp.	.3
Horseradish (French's)	1 tsp.	.3
Salad (French's) cream	1 tsp.	.3
Yellow (Gulden's)	1 tsp.	.4
MUSTARD GREENS (Birds Eye)	⅓ pkg.	3.0

N

Food and Description	Measure or Quantity	Carbohydrates (grams)
NATURAL CEREAL:		
(Heartland):		
Coconut	¼ cup	18.1
Coconut, hot	¼ cup	19.0
Plain oat or raisin	¼ cup	18.7
Regular or spice	¼ cup	19.0
Toasted corn	¼ cup	21.1
Toasted wheat	¼ cup	20.7
(Quaker) 100%	¼ cup	17.0
(Quaker) 100% with fruit	¼ cup	17.8
NEAPOLITAN ICE CREAM		
(Sealtest)	¼ pt.	18.0
NECTARINE, flesh only	4 oz.	19.4
NOODLE:		
Dry (Pennsylvania Dutch Brand) broad	1 oz.	20.0
Cooked, 1½″ strips	1 cup	37.3
NOODLES & BEEF, frozen (Banquet)	3-lb. pkg.	83.6
NOODLE, CHOW MEIN:		
(Chun King)	1 cup	23.2
(La Choy)	½ cup	15.8
(La Choy) wide	½ cup	16.0
NOODLE MIX:		
*(Betty Crocker):		
Almondine	¼ pkg.	27.0
Romanoff	¼ pkg.	23.0
Stroganoff	¼ pkg.	26.0
Noodle Roni, parmesano	⅛ of 6-oz. pkg.	23.2

Food and Description	Measure or Quantity	Carbohydrates (grams)
*(Pennsylvania Dutch Brand)		
Noodles Plus Sauce:		
Beef	½ cup	24.0
Butter	½ cup	23.0
Cheese	½ cup	24.0
Chicken	½ cup	25.0
*NOODLE, RAMEN (La Choy)		
canned:		
Beef	1 cup	33.4
Chicken	1 cup	29.1
Oriental	1 cup	30.7
NOODLE, RICE (La Choy)	1 oz.	19.9
NUT, MIXED:		
Dry roasted:		
(A&P)	1 oz.	6.6
(Flavor House)	1 oz.	5.4
(Planters)	1 oz.	7.0
Oil roasted:		
(Excel) with peanuts	1 oz.	5.4
(Planters) with peanuts	1 oz.	6.0
(Planters) without peanuts	1 oz.	6.0
NUTMEG (French's)	1 tsp.	.9
NUTRIMATO (Mott's)	6 fl. oz.	17.0

O

Food and Description	Measure or Quantity	Carbohydrates (grams)
OAT FLAKES, cereal (Post)	⅔ cup	20.1
OATMEAL:		
(H-O):		
Regular, dry, old fashioned	1 T.	3.0
Instant, dry	1 T.	2.8
Instant, dry, with raisins & spice	1 packet	32.9
Quick, dry	1 T.	2.8
(Quaker):		
Instant, dry	1-oz. packet	18.1
Instant, dry, bran & raisin	1½-oz. packet	29.2
Instant, dry, maple & brown sugar	1½-oz. packet	31.9
*(Ralston Purina) regular & quick	⅓ cup	9.0
(3-Minute Brand) *Stir'n Eat:*		
Dutch apple brown sugar	1⅛-oz. packet	23.3
Natural flavor	1-oz. packet	18.0
OCEAN PERCH:		
Fried	4 oz.	7.7
Frozen (Banquet)	8¾-oz. dinner	49.8
OIL, SALAD or COOKING:		
Crisco; Puritan	1 T.	0
Mazola, corn oil	1 T.	0
(Planters) peanut oil	1 T.	0
OKRA, frozen (Birds Eye) whole	⅓ pkg.	7.0

Food and Description	Measure or Quantity	Carbohydrates (grams)
OLD FASHIONED:		
Cocktail (Hiram Walker) 62 proof	3 fl. oz.	3.0
Dry mix (Bar-Tender's)	1 serving	4.7
OLIVE:		
Green	4 med. or 3 extra large or 2 giant	.2
Ripe, Mission	3 small or 2 large	.3
ONION:		
Raw	2½" onion	8.7
Boiled, pearl onions	½ cup	6.0
Canned (Durkee) O & C, boiled	¼ of 16-oz. jar	8.0
Canned (Durkee) O & C, creamed	¼ of 15½-oz. can	65.8
Dehydrated (Gilroy) flakes	1 tsp.	1.2
Frozen:		
(Birds Eye):		
Chopped	⅓ pkg.	2.0
Whole	⅓ pkg.	10.0
Creamed	⅓ pkg.	11.0
(Green Giant) creamed	⅛ pkg.	5.1
(Mrs. Paul's) french-fried rings	½ of 5-oz. pkg.	21.2
(Ore-Ida) chopped	2-oz. serving	4.0
(Ore-Ida) *Onion Ringers*	2-oz. serving	17.0
ONION BOUILLON:		
(Croyden House)	1 tsp.	2.3
(Herb-Ox)	1 cube	1.4
MBT	1 packet	2.0
ONION, GREEN	1 small onion	.9
ONION SOUP:		
Canned:		
(Campbell) condensed	10½-oz. can	18.9
*(Campbell) cream of	10-oz. serving	20.0
(Crosse & Blackwell)	½ of 13-oz. can	4.8
(Hormel)	½ of 15-oz. can	2.8
Mix:		
(Ann Page)	1⅜-oz. pkg.	21.1
*(Lipton)	1 cup	6.0
*(Lipton) beefy	1 cup	4.0
(Lipton) *Cup-a-Soup*	1 pkg.	5.0
*(Nestlé's) *Souptime*	6 fl. oz.	4.0
ORANGE:		
Peeled (Sunkist)	½ cup	16.0
Sections (Kraft)	4 oz.	9.0
ORANGEADE, chilled (Sealtest)	½ cup	8.0
ORANGE-APRICOT JUICE DRINK		
(Ann Page)	1 cup	31.2
ORANGE CREAM BAR (Sealtest)	2½-fl.-oz. bar	18.1
ORANGE DRINK:		
(Alegre) Island orange	8 fl. oz.	33.1
(Ann Page)	8 fl. oz.	30.2
(Hi-C)	8 fl. oz.	30.7
(Lincoln)	8 fl. oz.	31.9
*Mix (Hi-C)	8 fl. oz.	25.3

Food and Description	Measure or Quantity	Carbohydrates (grams)
ORANGE EXTRACT (Virginia Dare)	1 tsp.	0
ORANGE-GRAPEFRUIT JUICE:		
Bottled, chilled (Kraft)	½ cup	14.1
*Frozen (Minute Maid)	6 fl. oz.	19.1
ORANGE ICE (Sealtest)	¼ pt.	33.0
ORANGE JUICE:		
Fresh (Sunkist)	6 fl. oz.	19.5
Chilled (Kraft)	½ cup	13.8
Chilled (Sealtest)	½ cup	14.4
Canned (Del Monte) sweetened	6 fl. oz.	17.4
Canned, dietetic (Featherweight) unsweetened	½ cup	12.0
*Frozen (Minute Maid)	6 fl. oz.	21.4
ORANGE PEEL, candied (Liberty)	1 oz.	22.6
ORANGE-PINEAPPLE DRINK:		
(Ann Page)	1 cup	31.5
(Hi-C)	8 fl. oz.	30.7
(Lincoln)	8 fl. oz.	34.7
*ORANGE PLUS (Birds Eye)	6 fl. oz.	23.5
OREGANO (French's)	1 tsp.	1.0
OVALTINE, chocolate	¾ oz.	16.0
OYSTER:		
Raw:		
Eastern	19-31 small or 13-19 med.	8.2
Pacific & Western	6-9 small or 4-6 med.	15.4
Canned (Bumble Bee) solids & liq.	½ of 8-oz. can	5.5
Fried	4 oz.	21.1
OYSTER STEW:		
Home recipe	½ cup	5.7
*Soup (Campbell)	10-oz. serving	5.0

P

Food and Description	Measure or Quantity	Carbohydrates (grams)
PANCAKE, frozen with sausage (Swanson)	6-oz. breakfast	50.0
PANCAKE BATTER, frozen:		
*(Aunt Jemima):		
Plain and buttermilk	4" pancake	14.1
Blueberry	4" pancake	13.8
*(Rich's):		
Plain	1 pancake	17.9
Blueberry	⅒ of pkg.	16.5
Buttermilk	⅒ of pkg.	16.9
*PANCAKE & WAFFLE MIX:		
Plain:		
(Aunt Jemima) original	4" pancake	11.2
(Log Cabin) complete	4" pancake	8.7
(Pillsbury) Hungry Jack, complete	4" pancake	14.0

Food and Description	Measure or Quantity	Carbohydrates (grams)
(Pillsbury) *Hungry Jack Extra Lights*	4″ pancake	8.7
Blueberry (Pillsbury) *Hungry Jack*	4″ pancake	14.3
Buttermilk:		
(Aunt Jemima)	4″ pancake	13.3
(Aunt Jemima) complete	4″ pancake	15.4
(Betty Crocker) complete	4″ pancake	13.7
(Pillsbury) *Hungry Jack,* complete	4″ pancake	9.7
Whole wheat (Aunt Jemima)	4″ pancake	10.7
Dietetic (Tillie Lewis) complete	4″ pancake	8.6
PANCAKE & WAFFLE SYRUP:		
(Golden Griddle)	1 T.	13.4
Mrs. Butterworth's	1 T.	13.0
Dietetic (Diet Delight)	1 T.	.9
Dietetic (Featherweight)	1 T.	4.0
PAPAYA, fresh:		
Cubed	½ cup	9.1
Juice	4 oz.	18.8
PAPRIKA (French's)	1 tsp.	1.1
PARSLEY:		
Fresh, chopped	1 T.	.3
Dried (French's)	1 tsp.	.6
PASSION FRUIT, giant, whole	1 lb.	11.3
PASTINA (Ann Page)	1 oz.	20.5
PASTOSO (Petri)	3 fl. oz.	1.2
PASTRAMI (Vienna)	1 oz.	0
PASTRY SHELL:		
Pot pie (Keebler)	4″ shell	29.6
Tart (Keebler)	3″ shell	16.6
PÂTÉ:		
De foie gras	1 T.	.7
Liver (Sell's)	1 T.	.5
PDQ:		
Chocolate	1 T.	14.6
Strawberry	1 T.	15.1
PEA:		
Boiled	½ cup	9.9
Canned, solids & liq.:		
(April Showers) early	½ cup	10.6
(Del Monte) early	½ cup	9.9
(Del Monte) seasoned	½ cup	9.8
(Green Giant) early, with onions	½ cup	10.6
(Green Giant) sweet	½ cup	8.5
(Green Giant) *Sweetlets*	½ cup	8.2
(Green Giant) sweet, with onion	½ cup	8.5
(Kounty Kist) early	½ cup	12.8
(Kounty Kist) sweet	½ cup	8.5
(Le Sueur) early	½ cup	9.2
(Libby's) sweet	½ cup	11.6
(Lindy) sweet	½ cup	12.8
(Stokely-Van Camp) early	½ cup	12.5

Food and Description	Measure or Quantity	Carbohydrates (grams)
Canned, dietetic, solids & liq.:		
(Diet Delight)	½ cup	7.4
(Featherweight) sweet	½ cup	10.0
Frozen:		
(Birds Eye) cream sauce	⅓ pkg.	13.7
(Birds Eye) with sliced mushrooms	⅓ pkg.	10.7
(Birds Eye) sweet	⅓ pkg.	12.0
(Green Giant) creamed, *Bake 'n Serve*	⅓ pkg.	11.2
(Green Giant) early, small	4-oz. serving	12.5
(Green Giant) sweet	4½-oz. serving	14.1
(Green Giant) sweet, in butter sauce	⅓ pkg.	8.1
PEA & CARROT:		
Canned (Del Monte)	½ cup	9.4
Canned (Libby's)	½ cup	10.3
Canned, dietetic (Diet Delight)	½ cup	6.2
Frozen (Birds Eye)	⅓ pkg.	8.7
PEA & CAULIFLOWER, frozen (Birds Eye) creamed	⅓ pkg.	11.9
PEA & ONION, frozen (Birds Eye)	⅓ pkg.	11.7
PEA POD:		
Boiled, drained solids	4 oz.	10.8
Frozen (La Choy)	6-oz. pkg.	20.4
PEA & POTATO, frozen (Birds Eye), cream sauce	⅓ pkg.	16.3
PEA PUREE, canned, dietetic (Cellu)	½ cup	14.5
PEA SOUP, green:		
Canned:		
*(Campbell) condensed	8-oz. serving	23.2
Dietetic (Featherweight) low sodium	8-oz. can	32.0
*Mix:		
(Lipton)	1 cup	22.0
(Nestlé) *Souptime*	6 fl. oz.	14.0
PEA SOUP, split:		
*(Ann Page) with ham	1 cup	26.9
*(Campbell) with ham & bacon	8-oz. serving	24.0
(Campbell) with ham, *Chunky*	19-oz. can	60.0
PEACH:		
Fresh, with thin skin	2″ peach	9.6
Fresh, slices	½ cup	8.2
Canned:		
(Del Monte) Cling	½ cup	22.8
(Del Monte) spiced	½ cup	20.6
(Libby's) halves, heavy syrup, solids & liq.	½ cup	25.4
(Libby's) sliced, heavy syrup, solids & liq.	½ cup	24.7
(Stokely Van Camp)	½ cup	24.5

Food and Description	Measure or Quantity	Carbohydrates (grams)
Dietetic (Diet Delight)		
Cling, syrup pack, solids & liq.	½ cup	14.5
Dietetic (Diet Delight)		
Cling, water pack, solids & liq.	½ cup	7.0
Dried, canned (Del Monte)	2 oz.	35.2
Frozen (Birds Eye) sliced	5 oz.	34.1
PEACH BRANDY (DeKuyper)	1 fl. oz.	6.9
PEACH CREEK, wine		
(Annie Green Springs)	1 fl. oz.	2.3
PEACH DUMPLING (Pepperidge Farm)	1 piece	34.6
PEACH FRUIT DRINK (Hi-C):		
Canned	6 fl. oz.	23.0
*Mix	6 fl. oz.	19.0
PEACH ICE CREAM:		
(Breyer's)	¼ pt.	18.0
(Sealtest) old fashioned	¼ pt.	19.0
PEACH LIQUEUR (DeKuyper)	1 fl. oz.	8.3
PEACH PRESERVE:		
(Smucker's)	1 T.	13.1
Dietetic:		
(Dia-Mel; Louis Sherry)	1 tsp.	0
(Tillie Lewis)	1 tsp.	1.0
PEACH TURNOVER (Pepperidge Farm)	1 turnover	33.4
PEANUT:		
Dry (A&P)	1 oz.	5.7
Dry (Frito-Lay)	1 oz.	6.2
Dry (Planters)	1 oz.	5.4
Oil (Planters)	1 oz. (jar)	5.0
PEANUT BUTTER:		
(Ann Page) Krunchy or smooth	1 T.	3.6
(Bama) crunchy	1 T.	3.4
(Bama) smooth	1 T.	2.9
(Jif)	1 T.	2.7
(Peter Pan) smooth	1 T.	3.1
(Planters)	1 T.	2.7
(Skippy) creamy	1 T.	2.2
Dietetic (Cellu) low sodium	1 T.	2.2
PEANUT BUTTER BAKING CHIPS		
(Reese's)	3 T. (1 oz.)	12.8
PEANUT BUTTER PUDDING		
(Sanna)	3-oz. container	18.7
PEANUT SPREAD, *Koogle:*		
Banana, chocolate or vanilla	1 oz.	8.0
Cinnamon	1 oz.	7.0
PEAR:		
Whole	3" x 2½" pear	25.4
Canned:		
(Del Monte)	½ cup	21.3
(Libby's)	½ cup	25.1

Food and Description	Measure or Quantity	Carbohydrates (grams)
PEBBLES, cereal:		
Cocoa	⅞ cup	24.2
Fruity	⅞ cup	24.4
PECAN:		
Halves	6-7 pieces	1.0
Dry roasted (Flavor House)	1 oz.	4.1
Dry roasted (Planters)	1 oz.	5.0
PEP, cereal	¾ cup	24.0
PEPPER:		
Black (French's)	1 tsp.	1.5
Lemon (Durkee)	1 tsp.	.2
Seasoned (Lawry's)	1 tsp.	1.6
PEPPER, HOT CHILI:		
Canned (Ortega)	1 oz.	1.1
Dried (French's)	1 tsp.	1.2
PEPPER, STUFFED:		
Home recipe	2¾″ x 2½″ pepper with 1⅛ cups stuffing	31.1
Frozen:		
(Green Giant)	7-oz. serving	18.1
(Weight Watchers) with veal	12-oz. meal	51.0
PEPPER, SWEET:		
Green, whole	1 med.	2.9
Red, whole	1 med.	2.4
PEPPERONI (Swift)	1 oz.	1.0
***PEPPER POT SOUP (Campbell's)**	8-oz. serving	9.6
PERCH:		
White, meat only	4 oz.	0
Yellow, meat only	4 oz.	0
Frozen:		
(Banquet)	8¾-oz. dinner	49.8
(Mrs. Paul's) fillets, breaded & fried	2-oz. fillet	8.8
(Van de Kamp's) batter dipped, french fried	2.4-oz. piece	10.0
(Weight Watchers)	16-oz. meal	15.0
PERNOD (Julius Wile)	1 fl. oz.	1.1
PERSIMMON	4.4-oz. fruit	20.7
PICKLE:		
Cucumber, fresh or bread & butter (Aunt Jane's)	1 slice or stick	1.3
Dill:		
(Claussen) Kosher,	2-oz. serving	1.3
L & S	1 large pickle	2.0
(Smucker's) candied	4″ pickle	11.2
(Smucker's) Kosher	3½″ pickle	1.4
Sweet (Bond's) Gherkin	1 pickle	3.0
PIE:		
Apple:		
Home recipe, two crust	⅙ of 9″ pie	60.2
(Drake's)	2-oz. pie	25.5

Food and Description	*Measure or Quantity*	*Carbohydrates (grams)*
(Hostess)	4½-oz. pie	53.7
Banana, cream or custard, home recipe	⅙ of 9″ pie	46.7
Berry (Hostess)	4½-oz. pie	51.1
Blackberry, home recipe, two-crust	⅙ of 9″ pie	54.4
Blueberry, home recipe, two-crust	⅙ of 9″ pie	55.1
Blueberry (Hostess)	4½-oz. pie	49.9
Boston cream, home recipe	1/12 of 8″ pie	34.3
Cherry:		
Home recipe, two crust	⅙ of 9″ pie	60.7
(Hostess)	4½-oz. pie	58.8
Chocolate chiffon, home recipe	⅙ of 9″ pie	61.2
Chocolate meringue, home recipe	⅙ of 9″ pie	46.9
Coconut cream (Tastykake)	4-oz. pie	48.4
Coconut, custard, home recipe	⅙ of 9″ pie	37.8
Lemon (Hostess)	4½-oz. pie	52.4
Mince, home recipe, two-crust	⅙ of 9″ pie	65.1
Peach (Hostess)	4½-oz. pie	52.4
Pecan (Frito-Lay's)	3-oz. serving	53.5
Pumpkin, home recipe, one-crust	⅙ of 9″ pie	37.2
Raisin, home recipe, two-crust	⅙ of 9″ pie	67.9
Rhubarb, home recipe, two-crust	⅙ of 9″ pie	60.4
Frozen:		
Apple:		
(Banquet)	⅕ of 20-oz. pie	42.6
(Morton)	⅙ of 24-oz. pie	40.9
(Morton) mini	½ of 8-oz. pie	44.3
(Sara Lee)	5.2-oz. serving	50.2
(Sara Lee) Dutch	5-oz. serving	50.8
Banana:		
(Banquet) cream	⅙ of 14-oz. pie	19.9
(Morton) cream	⅙ of 16-oz. pie	19.7
(Morton) cream, mini	3½-oz. pie	25.8
Blueberry:		
(Banquet)	⅙ of 20-oz. pie	37.5
(Morton)	⅙ of 24-oz. pie	38.6
(Morton) mini	½ of 8-oz. pie	43.2
(Sara Lee)	5.2-oz. serving	50.8
Cherry:		
(Banquet)	⅙ of 20-oz. pie	33.8
(Morton)	⅙ of 24-oz. pie	42.0
(Morton) mini	½ of 8-oz. pie	43.2
(Sara Lee)	5.2-oz. serving	46.4
Chocolate cream:		
(Banquet)	⅙ of 14-oz. pie	21.8
(Morton)	⅙ of 16-oz. pie	22.8
(Morton) mini	3½-oz. pie	28.8
Coconut cream:		
(Banquet)	⅙ of 14-oz. pie	19.1
(Morton)	⅙ of 16-oz. pie	22.0
(Morton) mini	3½-oz. pie	28.8

Food and Description	*Measure or Quantity*	*Carbohydrates (grams)*
Coconut custard:		
(Banquet)	⅙ of 20-oz. pie	28.3
(Morton) mini	½ of 6½-oz. pie	26.8
Custard (Banquet)	⅕ of 20-oz. pie	38.1
Lemon cream:		
(Banquet)	⅙ of 14-oz. pie	21.8
(Morton)	⅙ of 16-oz. pie	22.0
(Morton) mini	3½-oz. pie	28.9
Mince:		
(Banquet)	⅙ of 20-oz. pie	38.5
(Morton)	⅙ of 24-oz. pie	45.5
(Morton) mini	½ of 8-oz. pie	46.6
Peach:		
(Banquet)	⅙ of 20-oz. pie	35.8
(Morton)	⅙ of 24-oz. pie	38.7
(Morton) mini	½ of 8-oz. pie	40.9
(Sara Lee)	⅙ of 31-oz. pie	54.3
Pecan (Morton) mini	½ of 6½-oz. pie	40.6
Pumpkin:		
(Banquet)	⅙ of 20-oz. pie	32.3
(Morton)	⅙ of 24-oz. pie	36.4
Strawberry cream (Banquet)	⅙ of 14-oz. pie	22.5
Mix:		
*Boston cream (Betty Crocker)	⅛ of pie	40.0
*Chocolate cream (Pillsbury) no bake	⅙ of pie	53.0
*Lemon chiffon (Pillsbury) no bake	⅙ of pie	50.0
*Vanilla marble (Pillsbury) no bake	⅙ of pie	49.0
***PIECRUST MIX** (Flako)	⅙ of 9" shell	29.0
PIE FILLING (See also **PUDDING** or **PIE FILLING**):		
Apple:		
(Comstock)	⅙ of 8" pie	28.5
(Wilderness)	21-oz. can	163.7
Apricot (Wilderness)	21-oz. can	176.7
Banana, cream (Comstock)	⅙ of 8" pie	22.1
Blackberry (Comstock)	1 cup	108.5
Blueberry (Lucky Leaf)	8-oz. serving	61.4
Cherry (Wilderness)	21-oz. can	168.3
Coconut custard, home recipe, made with egg yolk & milk	5 oz. (inc. crust)	41.3
Mincemeat (Wilderness)	¼ of 22-oz. can	65.1
Peach (Lucky Leaf)	8 oz.	74.0
Pumpkin (Del Monte)	1 cup	19.8
PIGS FEET, pickled (Hormel)	1-pint can	.2
PIMIENTO, drained (Ortega)	¼ cup	1.3
PIMM'S CUP, vodka (Julius Wile)	1 fl. oz.	1.8
PIÑA COLADA:		
(Party Tyme) 12½% alcohol	2 fl. oz.	5.1
Dry mix (Holland House)	1 serving	16.0

Food and Description	Measure or Quantity	Carbohydrates (grams)
Liquid mix (Holland House)	2 fl. oz.	30.0
PINEAPPLE:		
Fresh (Dole) chunks	½ cup	13.7
Canned:		
(Del Monte) slices, medium	½ cup	22.4
(Dole) slices	2 med. slices & 2½ T. juice	15.5
PINEAPPLE & GRAPEFRUIT DRINK (Wagner)	8 fl. oz.	28.8
PINEAPPLE JUICE:		
(Dole)	6-fl.-oz. can	22.8
(Stokely-Van Camp)	½ cup	15.5
*Frozen (Minute Maid)	6 fl. oz.	22.7
PINEAPPLE PRESERVE:		
Sweetened (Smucker's)	1 T.	13.7
Dietetic (Featherweight)	1 T.	4.0
PINE NUT, pignolias, shelled	1 oz.	3.3
PINK SQUIRREL COCKTAIL MIX (Holland House)	1 serving	17.0
PINOT CHARDONAY (Inglenook)	3 fl. oz.	.2
PISTACHIO NUT:		
In shell	½ cup	6.3
Shelled	¼ cup	5.9
PIZZA PIE:		
Home recipe	⅛ of 14″ pie	21.2
(Pizza Hut):		
Beef	½ of 10″ pie	55.0
Cheese	½ of 10″ pie	53.2
Pepperoni	½ of 10″ pie	54.4
Supreme	½ of 10″ pie	54.4
Frozen:		
Cheese:		
(Buitoni)	4 oz.	36.6
(Celeste)	½ of 7-oz. pie	31.8
(Celeste)	¼ of 19-oz. pie	36.2
(Jeno's)	½ of 13-oz. pie	54.0
(La Pizzeria)	¼ of 20-oz. pie	33.0
(La Pizzeria) thick crust	⅓ of 18½-oz. pie	46.0
Tostino's	½ of pie	53.0
(Weight Watchers)	6-oz. pie	37.2
Combination (La Pizzeria)	½ of 13½-oz. pie	43.0
Combination (La Pizzeria)	¼ of 24½-oz. pie	39.0
Combination, *Tostino's* classic	⅓ of pie	48.0
Combination (Van de Kamp's) thick crust	¼ of 23.4-oz. pie	24.0
Pepperoni:		
(Buitoni)	4 oz.	38.7
(Celeste)	¼ of 20-oz. pie	31.7
(Jeno's)	½ of 13-oz. pie	57.0
(La Pizzeria)	¼ of 21-oz. pie	42.0
Tostino's	½ of pie	52.0
(Van de Kamp's) thick crust	¼ of 22-oz. pie	38.0

Food and Description	Measure or Quantity	Carbohydrates (grams)
Sausage:		
(Buitoni)	4 oz.	34.1
(Celeste)	¼ of 22-oz. pie	33.9
(Jeno's) deluxe	⅓ of 21-oz. pie	53.0
(Kraft)	⅓ of 14½-oz. pie	33.2
(La Pizzeria)	½ of 13-oz. pie	41.0
Tostino's	½ of pie	54.0
Tostino's, deep crust	⅛ of pie	33.0
(Weight Watchers)	6-oz. pie	30.7
Sausage & mushroom (Celeste)	¼ of 24-oz. pie	34.3
PIZZA PIE MIX:		
Regular (Jeno's)	½ of pkg.	67.0
Cheese:		
(Jeno's)	½ of pkg.	62.0
*(Kraft)	4-oz. serving	26.1
Skillet Pizza (General Mills)	¼ pkg.	30.0
Pepperoni:		
(Jeno's)	½ of pkg.	67.0
Skillet Pizza (General Mills)	¼ of pkg.	31.0
Sausage:		
*(Kraft)	4-oz. serving	23.9
Skillet Pizza (General Mills)	¼ pkg.	29.0
PIZZA ROLL (Jeno's) 12 to pkg.:		
Cheeseburger	½-oz. roll	4.5
Pepperoni	½-oz. roll	4.2
Sausage	½-oz. roll	4.2
Shrimp & cheese	½-oz. roll	3.8
PIZZA SAUCE:		
(Contadina)	8 oz.	23.0
(Ragu)	5 oz.	15.0
PLUM:		
Fresh:		
Japanese & hybrid, fresh	2″ plum	6.9
Prune-type, fresh, halves	½ cup	15.8
Canned:		
(Stokely-Van Camp)	½ cup	30.0
Dietetic:		
(Cellu) water pack	½ cup	9.0
(Tillie Lewis) juice pack	½ cup	18.2
PLUM HOLLOW WINE		
(Annie Green Springs)	3 fl. oz.	6.8
PLUM JELLY, dietetic		
(Featherweight)	1 T.	4.0
PLUM PRESERVE (Smucker's)	1 T.	12.9
PLUM PUDDING (Richardson & Robbins)	¼ of 14½-oz. can	61.6
P.M. FRUIT DRINK (Mott's)	6 fl. oz.	22.0
POLISH-STYLE SAUSAGE (Vienna)	3-oz. piece	1.3
POLYNESIAN-STYLE DINNER (Swanson)	13-oz. dinner	65.0
POMEGRANATE, whole	1 lb.	41.7
POMMARD WINE (B&G)	3 fl. oz.	.4

Food and Description	Measure or Quantity	Carbohydrates (grams)
POPCORN:		
Plain (Jiffy Pop)	½ of 5-oz. pkg.	29.8
Buttered (Old London; Wise)	1 cup	6.4
Caramel-coated:		
(Bachman)	1 oz.	23.0
(Old London) without peanuts	1¾-oz. bag	43.6
(Old London) with peanuts	1 cup	30.2
(Old London; Wise) with cheese	¾-oz. bag	6.6
Cheese flavored (Bachman)	1 oz.	14.0
Cracker Jack	¾-oz. bag	16.7
***POPOVER MIX** (Flako)	1 popover	25.0
POPPY SEED (French's)	1 tsp.	.8
POP TARTS (Kellogg's) regular	1.8-oz. pastry	36.0
PORK:		
Fresh:	Any quantity	0
Loin:	Any quantity	0
Cured ham:	Any quantity	0
(Hormel) picnic, canned	4 oz.	.2
(Wilson) Festival, smoked	4 oz.	1.0
PORK DINNER (Swanson)	11¼-oz. dinner	48.0
PORK RINDS, *Baken-ets*	1 oz.	.5
PORK SAUSAGE, cooked (Oscar Mayer) *Little Friers*	1 link	.5
PORK, SWEET & SOUR, frozen:		
(Chun King)	½ of 15-oz. pkg.	26.0
(La Choy)	½ of 15-oz. entree	45.2
PORT WINE:		
(Gallo)	3 fl. oz.	7.8
(Great Western) Solera	3 fl. oz.	11.5
(Louis M. Martini)	3 fl. oz.	2.0
****POSTUM***, instant	6 fl. oz.	2.0
POTATO:		
Cooked:		
Au gratin	½ cup	17.9
Baked, peeled	2½" dia. potato	20.9
Boiled, peeled	4.3-oz. potato	17.7
French-fried	10 pieces	20.5
Hash-browned, home recipe	½ cup	28.4
Mashed, milk & butter added	½ cup	12.1
Canned (Del Monte) drained	1 cup	28.4
Dehydrated (Borden) mashed	¼ cup	13.3
Frozen:		
(Birds Eye):		
Cottage fries	⅕ of 14-oz. pkg.	17.0
Crinkle cuts	3-oz. serving	18.4
French-fries	3-oz. serving	16.8
Tasti Puffs	¼ of 10-oz. pkg.	18.0
Tiny Taters	⅕ of 16-oz. pkg.	22.0
(Green Giant):		
Au gratin, *Bake 'n Serve*	⅓ of 10-oz. pkg.	12.1

Food and Description	Measure or Quantity	Carbohydrates (grams)
Diced, in sour cream sauce	1 cup	36.0
Stuffed with cheese-flavored topping	5-oz. entree	30.0
(Ore-Ida):		
Cottage fries	3.2-oz. serving	23.5
Country Style Dinner Fries	3-oz. serving	18.0
Crispers	3.2-oz. serving	27.7
Golden Crinkles	3.2-oz. serving	21.0
Golden Fries	3.2-oz. serving	23.4
Hash browns, shredded	6-oz. serving	24.0
Hash browns, Southern style	3.2-oz. serving	17.1
Hash browns, Southern style, with butter sauce	3-oz. serving	15.0
Hash browns, Southern style, with butter sauce & onions	3-oz. serving	17.0
O'Brien potatoes	3-oz. serving	14.0
Pixie Crinkles	3.3-oz. serving	27.5
Shoestrings	3.3-oz. serving	27.5
Tater Tots, plain	3.2-oz. serving	21.3
Tater Tots, bacon flavor	3.2-oz. serving	22.4
Tater Tots, with onion	3.2-oz. serving	22.4
Whole, small, peeled	3.2-oz. serving	17.1
POTATO CHIP:		
(Bachman)	1 oz.	14.0
(Frito-Lay; Pringle's; *Ruffles*)	1 oz.	15.1
Lay's	1 oz.	14.0
Lay's, sour cream & onion flavor	1 oz.	14.7
(Planters) stackable	1 oz.	17.0
(Wise)	1 oz.	15.7
(Wise) barbecue flavor	1 oz.	15.8
(Wise) onion & garlic	1 oz.	15.1
***POTATO MIX:**		
Au gratin:		
(Betty Crocker)	⅙ pkg.	20.0
(French's)	½ cup	28.6
Buds (Betty Crocker)	⅓ cup	15.0
Julienne (Betty Crocker)	⅙ pkg.	17.0
Mashed:		
(French's) *Big Tate*	½ cup	16.0
(Pillsbury) *Hungry Jack*, flakes	½ cup (4 to pkg.)	18.0
Scalloped:		
(Betty Crocker)	⅙ pkg.	20.0
(French's)	½ cup	30.0
POTATO PANCAKE MIX		
(French's) *Big Tate*	3″ pancake	5.7
POTATO SALAD, home recipe	½ cup	16.8
***POTATO SOUP** (Campbell)	10-oz. serving	14.0
POTATO STICK:		
O & C (Durkee)	1½-oz. can	22.0
(Wise) French fries	1 oz.	19.3

Food and Description	Measure or Quantity	Carbohydrates (grams)
(Wise) Julienne	1-oz. pkg.	15.2
POUILLY-FUISSÉ WINE:		
(B&G)	3 fl. oz.	.3
(Canson) St. Vincent	3 fl. oz.	6.3
POUND CAKE (See CAKE, Pound)		
PRESERVES:		
(Ann Page) all flavors	2 tsps.	9.6
(Crosse & Blackwell)	1 T.	14.8
PRETZEL:		
(Bachman):		
Thins	1 oz.	22.0
Nutzel	1 oz.	21.0
(Nabisco) *Mister Salty*, pretzelette	½-oz. piece	1.3
(Old London; Wise) nuggets	1 oz.	22.5
Rold Gold, twists	1 oz.	21.7
(Wise):		
Old fashioned	1 oz.	21.3
Rods	1 oz.	22.2
Sticks	1 oz.	22.7
Thins	1 oz.	22.2
PRODUCT 19, cereal (Kellogg's)	1 oz.	24.0
PRUNE:		
Dried, cooked	8 prunes & 5 T. liq.	66.1
Canned (Sunsweet)	5-6 prunes	32.9
Canned, dietetic (Featherweight) stewed, water pack	½ cup	35.0
PRUNE JUICE:		
(Ann Page)	½ cup	22.4
(Mott's)	6 fl. oz.	34.0
PRUNE WHIP, home recipe	½ cup	24.9
PUDDING or PIE FILLING:		
Canned, regular pack:		
Banana (Del Monte)	5-oz. container	30.1
Butterscotch (Del Monte)	5-oz. container	30.8
Butterscotch (Thank You)	½ cup	29.2
Chocolate:		
(Betty Crocker)	5-oz. serving	30.0
(Del Monte)	5-oz. container	33.0
(Thank You)	½ cup	29.2
Lemon (Thank You)	½ cup	36.2
Rice:		
(Comstock)	½ cup	24.5
(Betty Crocker)	½ cup	25.0
Tapioca:		
(Betty Crocker)	½ cup	22.0
(Del Monte)	5-oz. container	30.1
Vanilla:		
(Betty Crocker)	5-oz. serving	29.0
(Del Monte)	5-oz. container	32.1
Canned, dietetic (Sego) all flavors	½ of 8-oz. container	19.5
Chilled or refrigerated,		

Food and Description	Measure or Quantity	Carbohydrates (grams)
Swiss Miss:		
Butterscotch	4½-oz. container	23.0
Chocolate	4¼-oz. container	28.0
Tapioca	4½-oz. container	24.0
Vanilla	4¼-oz. container	26.0
Frozen (Rich's):		
Banana	3-oz. container	19.3
Butterscotch	4½-oz. container	27.4
Chocolate	4½-oz. container	27.1
Vanilla	4½-oz. container	27.5
Mix, sweetened, regular & instant:		
Banana:		
(Ann Page) regular	¼ of 3⅛-oz. pkg.	21.0
*(Jell-O) regular	⅙ of 8" pie, excluding crust	18.0
*(Jell-O) cream, instant	½ cup	13.0
*(Royal) regular	½ cup	27.0
*(Royal) instant	½ cup	29.0
*Butter pecan (Jell-O) instant	½ cup	29.0
Butterscotch:		
(Ann Page) regular	¼ of 3⅝-oz. pkg.	24.1
*(Jell-O) regular or instant	½ cup	30.0
*(My-T-Fine) regular	½ cup	38.0
*(Royal) regular	½ cup	27.0
*(Royal) instant	½ cup	29.0
Chocolate:		
(Ann Page) regular	¼ of 3⅝-oz. pkg.	23.7
*(Jell-O) regular	½ cup	29.0
*(Jell-O) instant	½ cup	34.0
*(My-T-Fine) regular	½ cup	27.0
*(My-T-Fine) regular, fudge	½ cup	27.0
*(Royal) regular	½ cup	33.0
*(Royal) instant	½ cup	35.0
Coconut:		
(Ann Page)	¼ of 3½-oz. pkg.	18.1
*(Jell-O) cream, regular	⅙ of 8" pie, excluding crust	17.0
*(Royal) instant	½ cup	30.0
*Coffee (Royal) instant	½ cup	29.0
Custard:		
(Ann Page) egg, regular	¼ of 2¾-oz. pkg.	15.4
*Jell-O Americana, golden egg	½ cup	24.0
*(Royal) regular	½ cup	22.0
*Flan (Royal) regular	½ cup	22.0
Lemon:		
(Ann Page) regular	¼ of 3-oz. pkg.	20.0
*(Jell-O) instant	½ cup	31.0
*(My-T-Fine) regular	½ cup	30.0
*(Royal) regular	½ cup	30.0
*(Royal) instant	½ cup	29.0

Food and Description	Measure or Quantity	Carbohydrates (grams)
*Lime (Royal) Key Lime, regular	½ cup	30.0
*Pineapple (Jell-O) cream, instant	½ cup	31.0
Pistachio:		
(Ann Page) instant	¼ of 3½-oz. pkg.	22.7
*(Jell-O) instant	½ cup	30.0
*(Royal) nut, instant	½ cup	30.0
*Rice, *Jell-O Americana*	½ cup	30.0
Tapioca:		
Jell-O Americana, chocolate or vanilla	½ cup	27.0
*(My-T-Fine) vanilla	½ cup	28.0
*(Royal) chocolate	½ cup	33.0
*(Royal) vanilla	½ cup	27.0
Vanilla:		
*(Jell-O) regular	½ cup	27.0
*(Jell-O) French, regular & instant	½ cup	30.0
*(My-T-Fine) regular	½ cup	28.0
*(Royal) regular	½ cup	27.0
*(Royal) instant	½ cup	29.0
Mix, dietetic:		
*Butterscotch:		
(D-Zerta)	½ cup	13.0
(Featherweight)	4-oz. serving	10.0
(Featherweight) artificially sweetened	4-oz. serving	3.0
*Chocolate:		
(Dia-Mel)	4-oz. serving	8.2
(D-Zerta)	½ cup	12.0
(Estee)	½ cup	16.0
(Featherweight)	4-oz. serving	9.0
(Featherweight) artificially sweetened	4-oz. serving	2.0
*Custard (Featherweight)	4-oz. serving	9.0
*Lemon (Dia-Mel)	½ cup	8.2
*Vanilla:		
(D-Zerta)	½ cup	13.0
(Estee)	½ cup	16.0
(Featherweight)	4-oz. serving	10.0
(Featherweight) artificially sweetened	4-oz. serving	3.0
PUFFED RICE, cereal:		
(Malt-O-Meal)	½ oz.	11.9
(Quaker)	1 cup	12.7
PUFFED WHEAT, cereal:		
(Malt-O-Meal)	½ oz.	9.9
(Quaker)	1 cup	10.8
PUFFS, frozen (Rich's) vanilla	1 puff	23.4
PULIGNY MONTRACHET WINE:		
(B&G)	3 fl. oz.	.3

Food and Description	Measure or Quantity	Carbohydrates (grams)
(Chanson)	3 fl. oz.	6.3
PUMPKIN SEED, in hull	1 oz.	3.2

Q

QUAIL, raw, meat & skin	4 oz.	0
QUIK (Nestlé):		
Chocolate	3 heaping tsps.	19.0
Strawberry	3 heaping tsps.	21.0
QUINCE JELLY (Smucker's)	1 T.	13.1
QUISP, cereal	1⅛ cups	23.1

R

RADISH	2 small radishes	.7
RAISIN (Del Monte)	3 oz.	66.5
RALSTON, cereal	¼ cup	20.0
RASPBERRY:		
Fresh, trimmed, black	½ cup	10.5
Fresh, trimmed, red	½ cup	9.8
Frozen (Birds Eye) quick thaw	5-oz. serving	34.8
RASPBERRY BRANDY (DeKuyper)	1 fl. oz.	6.9
RASPBERRY DRINK MIX (Wyler's)	3-oz. pouch	84.6
RASPBERRY PRESERVE:		
Sweetened (Smucker's)	1 T.	13.7
Dietetic (Dia-Mel) black	1 T.	0
Dietetic (Featherweight)	1 T.	4.0
RASPBERRY SYRUP (Smucker's)	1 T.	11.1
RASPBERRY TURNOVER (Pepperidge Farm)	1 turnover	36.9
RAVIOLI:		
Canned:		
(Franco-American) beef, *Raviolios*	½ of 15-oz. can	32.0
(Prince) cheese	3.7-oz. can	18.5
(Prince) meat	3.7-oz. can	18.7
Dietetic (Dia-Mel; Featherweight) beef, in sauce	8-oz. can	35.0
Frozen (Buitoni)	4 oz.	48.6
RELISH:		
Barbecue (Crosse & Blackwell)	1 T.	5.4
Corn (Crosse & Blackwell)	1 T.	3.6
RHINESKELLER WINE (Italian Swiss Colony)	3 fl. oz.	3.0
RHINE WINE:		
(Great Western)	3 fl. oz.	2.9
(Inglenook) Navelle	3 fl. oz.	4.3
(Italian Swiss Colony)	3 fl. oz.	1.2
(Taylor)	3 fl. oz.	3.0

Food and Description	*Measure or Quantity*	*Carbohydrates (grams)*
RHUBARB, cooked, sweetened	½ cup	43.2
RICE:		
*Brown (Uncle Ben's) parboiled, added butter	⅔ cup	26.4
White:		
*(Minute Rice) instant, no added butter	⅔ cup	27.0
*(Success) long grain	½ cooking bag	23.0
Mix (see **RICE MIX**)		
RICE CHEX, cereal	1⅛ cups	23.0
RICE, FRIED:		
*Canned (La Choy):		
Chicken	½ cup	40.1
Chinese style	½ cup	42.8
Frozen:		
(La Choy) & pork	½ of 12-oz. entree	38.8
(Temple) & shrimp	1 cup	51.0
***RICE, FRIED, SEASONING MIX** (Durkee)	1 cup	46.5
RICE KRINKLES, cereal	⅞ cup	26.3
RICE KRISPIES, cereal	1 cup	25.0
RICE MIX:		
Beef:		
(Ann Page) *Rice 'n Easy*	⅙ pkg.	26.2
*(Carolina) *Bake-It-Easy*	⅙ of 6-oz. pkg.	23.0
Rice-A-Roni	⅙ of 8-oz. pkg.	27.0
Chicken:		
(Ann Page) *Rice 'n Easy*	⅙ pkg.	27.4
*(Carolina) *Bake-It-Easy*	⅙ of 6-oz. pkg.	23.0
Rice-A-Roni	⅕ of 8-oz. pkg.	33.2
*Drumstick (Minute Rice)	½ cup	25.0
*Fried (Minute Rice)	½ cup	25.0
*Long grain & wild (Uncle Ben's) with butter	½ cup	20.6
*Oriental (Carolina) *Bake-It-Easy*	⅙ pkg.	25.0
*Rib roast (Minute Rice)	½ cup	25.0
Spanish:		
*(Carolina) *Bake-It-Easy*	⅙ of 6-oz. pkg.	24.0
*(Minute Rice)	½ cup	25.0
Rice-A-Roni	⅙ of 7½-oz. pkg.	25.9
RICE, SPANISH, canned:		
(Libby's)	7½-oz. serving	27.5
(Van Camp)	½ cup	15.5
Dietetic (Featherweight)	½ of 7¼-oz. can	14.0
***RICE, SPANISH, SEASONING MIX** (Durkee)	1 cup	44.7
RICE & VEGETABLES, frozen:		
(Birds Eye) with peas & mushrooms	⅓ pkg.	22.4
(Green Giant):		
& broccoli in cheese sauce	½ of 11-oz. pkg.	22.7

Food and Description	Measure or Quantity	Carbohydrates (grams)
Continental, with green bean & almonds	½ of 11-oz. pkg.	21.4
Medley, with peas & mushrooms	½ of 11-oz. pkg.	23.7
Pilaf, with mushrooms & onions	½ of 11-oz. pkg.	28.7
Verdi, with bell pepper & parsley	½ of 11-oz. pkg.	32.0
RICE WINE:		
Chinese, 20.7% alcohol	1 fl. oz.	1.1
Japanese, 10.6% alcohol	1 fl. oz.	13.1
Non-alcoholic	1 oz.	6.6
RIESLING WINE, Grey (Inglenook)	3 fl. oz.	.7
RING DINGS (Drake's):		
Jr., dark chocolate	2½-oz. piece	40.0
Jr., milk chocolate	2½-oz. piece	43.1
Restaurant size	2-oz. piece	31.5
ROCKFISH, steamed	4 oz.	2.2
ROCK & RYE (Garnier)	1 fl. oz.	6.2
ROE, baked or broiled, cod & shad	4 oz.	2.2
ROLAIDS	1 piece	1.4
ROLL & BUN:		
Apple crunch (Sara Lee)	1 roll	13.5
Biscuit (Wonder)	1 roll	34.0
Brown & serve (Wonder) *Gem Style*	1 roll	13.6
Butter crescent (Pepperidge Farm)	1 roll	13.0
Caramel pecan (Sara Lee)	1 roll	14.6
Caramel sticky (Sara Lee)	1 roll	15.0
Cinnamon (Sara Lee)	1 roll	12.6
Club (Pepperidge Farm)	1 roll	20.0
Croissant (Sara Lee)	1 roll	11.2
Deli Twist (Arnold)	1 roll	17.0
Dinner:		
(Arnold)	1 roll	9.5
(Pepperidge Farm)	1 roll	10.0
(Wonder)	1 roll	34.0
Finger:		
(Arnold) *Dinner Party*	1 roll	10.0
(Pepperidge Farm) poppy	1 roll	8.0
(Pepperidge Farm) sesame	1 roll	8.7
Frankfurter:		
(Arnold) hot dog	1 roll	20.0
(Wonder)	2-oz. roll	29.0
French:		
(Arnold) *Francisco,* sourdough	1 roll	19.0
(Pepperidge Farm) small	1 roll	48.0
(Pepperidge Farm) large	1 roll	76.0
Golden Twist (Pepperidge Farm)	1 roll	14.0
Hamburger:		
(Arnold)	1 roll	21.0
(Pepperidge Farm)	1 roll	19.0
(Wonder)	2-oz. roll	29.0
Hard (Levy's)	1 roll	37.4
Hearth (Pepperidge Farm)	1 roll	10.0

Food and Description	Measure or Quantity	Carbohydrates (grams)
Honey (Hostess)	1 cake	63.4
Honey (Sara Lee)	1 roll	14.6
Kaiser-Hogie (Wonder)	1 roll	82.0
Old fashioned (Pepperidge Farm)	1 roll	7.7
Parker house:		
(Arnold) *Dinner Party*	1 roll	10.0
(Pepperidge Farm)	1 roll	9.0
(Sara Lee)	1 roll	10.3
Party (Sara Lee)	1 roll	7.7
Party Pan (Pepperidge Farm)	1 roll	5.2
Poppy seed (Sara Lee)	1 roll	7.7
Sandwich (Arnold) soft	1 roll	18.0
Sesame Crisp (Pepperidge Farm)	1 roll	12.3
Sesame seed (Sara Lee)	1 roll	7.7
Tea (Arnold) *Dinner Party*	1 roll	6.0
ROLL DOUGH:		
*Frozen (Rich's) onion	2½-oz. roll	36.7
Refrigerated (Pillsbury):		
Caramel bun	1 bun	19.0
Cinnamon, with icing	1 bun	17.5
Dinner, crescent	1 roll	12.5
*ROLL MIX (Pillsbury) hot	1 roll	15.5
ROSEMARY LEAVES (French's)	1 tsp.	.8
ROSÉ WINE:		
(Antinori, Chanson)	3 fl. oz.	6.3
(Great Western)	3 fl. oz.	2.4
(Inglenook) Gamay or Vintage	3 fl. oz.	.5
(Mogen David)	3 fl. oz.	8.9
RUM & COLA (Party Tyme) 10% alcohol	2 fl. oz.	5.2
RUTABAGA, boiled, diced	½ cup	7.1

S

Food and Description	Measure or Quantity	Carbohydrates (grams)
SAFFLOWER SEED, in hull	1 oz.	1.8
SAGE (French's)	1 tsp.	.6
SAINT-EMILION WINE (B&G)	3 fl. oz.	.7
SAKE WINE	1 fl. oz.	1.4
SALAD DRESSING:		
Regular:		
Avocado Goddess (Marie's)	1 T.	1.0
Bacon (Marie's)	1 T.	1.0
Bleu or blue cheese:		
(Kraft) *Imperial*	1 T.	.9
(Marie's)	1 T.	1.0
(Wish-Bone) chunky	1 T.	1.0
Caesar:		
(Lawry's)	1 T.	.5
(Pfeiffer)	1 T.	.5
(Wish-Bone)	1 T.	1.0
Coleslaw (Kraft)	1 T.	3.6

Food and Description	Measure or Quantity	Carbohydrates (grams)
French:		
(Bernstein's)	1 T.	1.5
(Kraft) *Catalina*	1 T.	3.7
(Pfeiffer)	1 T.	3.5
(Wish-Bone) Deluxe	1 T.	2.0
Garlic (Wish-Bone) creamy	1 T.	1.0
German style (Marzetti)	1 T.	2.4
Green Goddess:		
(Bernstein's)	1 T.	1.1
(Kraft)	1 T.	.8
(Wish-Bone)	1 T.	1.0
Green onion (Kraft)	1 T.	1.1
Italian:		
(Kraft)	1 T.	1.1
(Lawry's) with cheese	1 T.	4.7
(Marie's)	1 T.	1.1
(Pfeiffer) chef	1 T.	.5
(Wish-Bone)	1 T.	1.0
Miracle Whip (Kraft)	1 T.	1.8
Oil & vinegar (Kraft)	1 T.	.6
Onion (Marie's) creamy	1 T.	1.4
Onion (Wish-Bone) California	1 T.	1.0
Ranch (Marie's)	1 T.	1.3
Roquefort:		
(Kraft)	1 T.	.8
(Marie's)	1 T.	1.1
Royal Scandia (Bernstein's)	1 T.	1.1
Russian:		
(Kraft)	1 T.	4.3
(Kraft) with pure honey	1 T.	4.6
(Pfeiffer)	1 T.	2.0
(Wish-Bone)	1 T.	7.0
Saffola	1 T.	2.2
Sesame (Sahadi) creamy	1 T.	2.0
Sesame (Sahadi) spice	1 T.	1.0
Spin Blend (Hellmann's)	1 T.	2.7
Sweet 'N' Sour (Dutch Pantry) creamy	1 T.	4.0
Thousand Island:		
(Kraft)	1 T.	2.5
(Marie's)	1 T.	1.6
(Pfeiffer)	1 T.	2.0
Vinaigrette (Bernstein's)	1 T.	.8
Dietetic:		
Bleu or blue cheese:		
(Ann Page)	1 T.	.5
(Dia-Mel)	1 T.	0
(Featherweight)	1 T.	1.0
Caesar (Dia-Mel)	1 T.	.5
Caesar (Pfeiffer)	1 T.	1.0
Chef style (Ann Page)	1 T.	3.2

Food and Description	Measure or Quantity	Carbohydrates (grams)
Chef's (Tillie Lewis)	1 T.	.4
Cucumber & onion (Featherweight) creamy	1 T.	0
French:		
(Cellu) low sodium	1 T.	0
(Dia-Mel)	1 T.	1.0
(Diet Delight)	1 T.	.8
(Featherweight) imitation	1 T.	1.0
(Kraft)	1 T.	2.0
(Pfeiffer)	1 T.	2.5
(Wish-Bone)	1 T.	4.0
Imitation (Featherweight)	1 T.	1.0
Italian:		
(Ann Page) creamy	1 T.	.7
(Dia-Mel; Tillie Lewis)	1 T.	.5
(Featherweight) creamy	1 T.	0
(Kraft)	1 T.	.6
(Pfeiffer)	1 T.	1.5
(Weight Watchers)	1 T.	2.0
(Wish-Bone)	1 T.	1.0
May-Lo-Naise (Tillie Lewis)	1 T.	1.0
Mayolite (Diet Delight)	1 T.	.7
Red wine (Pfeiffer)	1 T.	1.0
Russian:		
(Dia-Mel)	1 T.	.5
(Featherweight)	1 T.	1.0
(Kraft)	1 T.	4.3
(Pfeiffer)	1 T.	2.0
(Weight Watchers)	1 T.	2.0
(Wish-Bone)	1 T.	5.0
Soyamaise (Cellu) low sodium	1 T.	0
Thousand Island:		
(Dia-Mel)	1 T.	1.0
(Diet Delight)	1 T.	.5
(Featherweight)	1 T.	1.1
(Pfeiffer)	1 T.	2.0
(Weight Watchers)	1 T.	2.0
(Wish-Bone)	1 T.	3.0
2-Calorie Low Sodium (Featherweight)	1 T.	0
Whipped (Dia-Mel)	1 T.	2.1
Whipped (Tillie Lewis)	1 T.	1.0
SALAD DRESSING MIX:		
Regular:		
Bacon (Lawry's)	1 pkg.	11.9
Bleu or blue cheese:		
*(Good Seasons)	1 T.	.5
*(Good Seasons) *Thick 'n Creamy*	1 T.	.5
(Lawry's)	1 pkg.	4.5
*Buttermilk Farm Style (Good Seasons)	1 T.	1.0

Food and Description	Measure or Quantity	Carbohydrates (grams)
French:		
*(Good Seasons) old fashion	1 T.	1.0
*(Good Seasons) *Thick 'n Creamy*	1 T.	2.0
*Garlic (Good Seasons)	1 T.	1.0
Italian:		
*(Good Seasons)	1 T.	1.0
*Onion (Good Seasons)	1 T.	1.0
*Thousand Island (Good Seasons) *Thick 'n Creamy*	1 T.	2.0
Dietetic:		
French (Dia-Mel; Louis Sherry)	½ pkg.	0
Garlic (Dia-Mel)	½-oz. packet	1.0
Italian (Dia-Mel; Louis Sherry)	½-oz. packet	0
*Italian (Good Seasons)	1 T.	2.0
Russian (Louis Sherry)	½-oz. packet	0
Thousand Island (Dia-Mel)	½-oz. packet	0
SALAD FIXIN'S **(Arnold):**		
Danish-style blue cheese or French onion	½ oz.	8.8
Spicy Italian	½ oz.	8.7
SALAMI:		
(Oscar Mayer):		
For beer	.8-oz. slice	.3
Cotto	.8-oz. slice	.6
Cotto, beef	1-oz. slice	.6
Hard, all meat	.3-oz. slice	.1
(Swift) Genoa	1 oz.	.3
(Vienna) beef	1 oz.	.8
SALISBURY STEAK:		
Canned (Morton House)	⅓ of 12½-oz. can	7.0
Frozen:		
(Banquet) buffet	2-lb. pkg.	48.2
(Banquet) *Man Pleaser*	19-oz. dinner	71.7
(Green Giant) with gravy, oven bake	7-oz. entree	14.0
(Green Giant) with tomato sauce	9-oz. entree	22.0
(Morton)	11-oz. dinner	25.1
(Morton) *Country Table*	15-oz. dinner	51.1
(Swanson)	11½-oz. dinner	40.0
(Swanson) 3-course	16-oz. dinner	48.0
(Swanson) *Hungry Man*	17-oz. dinner	65.0
SALMON:		
Baked or broiled	6¾" x 2½" x 1"	0
Canned:		
Pink or Humpback:		
(Del Monte)	7¾-oz. can	0
(Icy Point; Pink Beauty)	7¾-oz. can	0
Sockeye or Red or Blueback:		
(Bumble Bee) solids & liq.	7¾-oz. can	0
(Del Monte)	7¾-oz. can	0
(Icy Point; Pillar Rock)	3¾-oz. can	0

Food and Description	Measure or Quantity	Carbohydrates (grams)
SALMON, SMOKED (Vita):		
Lox, drained	4-oz. jar	.2
Nova, drained	4-oz. can	1.0
SALT:		
(Morton) *Lite Salt*	1 tsp.	0
(Morton) table	1 tsp.	0
Substitute:		
(Adolph's) plain	1 tsp.	Tr.
(Adolph's) seasoned	1 tsp.	1.1
(Morton) plain	1 tsp.	Tr.
Salt-It (Dia-Mel)	1 tsp.	0
SANDWICH SPREAD:		
(Best Foods; Hellmann's)	1 T.	2.2
(Kraft) Pimiento	1 oz.	.8
SANGRIA (Taylor)	3 fl. oz.	10.8
SARDINE:		
Atlantic, canned (Del Monte)		
with tomato sauce	7½-oz. can	4.0
Norwegian, canned (Underwood):		
In mustard sauce	3¾-oz. can	2.3
In oil, drained	3¾-oz. can	.4
In tomato sauce	3¾-oz. can	4.5
SAUCE:		
A-1	1 T.	2.8
Barbecue:		
Chris & Pitt's	1 T.	4.0
(French's)	1 T.	3.0
(Kraft) hickory smoke	1 oz.	7.9
Open Pit (General Foods)		
hickory smoke	1 T.	4.0
Open Pit (General Foods)		
with minced onion	1 T.	4.0
Cocktail (Pfeiffer)	1-oz. serving	12.0
Escoffier Sauce Diable	1 T.	4.2
Escoffier Sauce Robert	1 T.	4.5
Famous (Durkee)	1 T.	2.2
Horseradish (Marzetti)	1 T.	2.3
Hot, *Frank's*	1 tsp.	2.0
H.P. Steak Sauce (Lee & Perrin)	1 T.	4.8
Italian (Carnation)	2 fl. oz.	7.0
Italian (Ragu) red cooking	3½ oz.	6.0
Marinara (Ragu)	5 oz.	15.0
Newburg (Snow)	½ cup	14.6
Seafood (Bernstein's)	1 T.	4.6
Seafood cocktail (Del Monte)	1 T.	4.9
Soy (Kikkoman)	1 T.	1.1
Soy (La Choy)	1 T.	.9
Steak (Dawn Fresh) with		
mushrooms	2-oz. serving	3.5
Steak Supreme	1 T.	4.8
Sweet & sour (Carnation)	1 T.	16.0
Sweet & Sour (La Choy)	1 oz.	12.6

Food and Description	Measure or Quantity	Carbohydrates (grams)
Swiss Steak (Carnation)	2-oz. serving	4.5
Taco (Ortega)	1 T.	4.8
Tartar (Best Foods; Hellmann's)	1 T.	.2
Teriyaki (Kikkoman)	1 T.	2.8
White, medium	¼ cup	5.6
Worcestershire (Lea & Perrin)	1 T.	3.0
SAUCE MIX:		
A la king (Durkee)	1 pkg.	14.0
*Cheese (Durkee)	¼ cup	4.8
Cheese (French's)	1 pkg.	14.0
Hollandaise (Durkee)	1 pkg.	11.0
Sour cream (French's)	1 pkg.	16.0
SAUERKRAUT:		
(Claussen) drained solids	¼ of 32-oz. jar	8.9
(Del Monte) solids & liq.	1 cup	10.7
(Libby's) solids & liq.	8-oz. can	9.6
(Stokely-Van Camp) Bavarian style, solids & liq.	½ cup	7.0
SAUSAGE:		
Beef, *Cow-Boy Jo's*	⅝ oz.	.9
Breakfast (Oscar Mayer)	.7-oz. link	.3
Brown & serve (Swift) original	1 cooked link	.5
*Patties (Oscar Mayer)	1 cooked pattie	0
SAUTERNE:		
(B&G)	3 fl. oz.	7.6
(Great Western)	3 fl. oz.	4.5
(Italian Swiss Colony)	3 fl. oz.	1.2
(Taylor)	3 fl. oz.	4.8
SAVORY (French's)	1 tsp.	1.0
SCALLOP:		
Steamed	4 oz.	DNA
Frozen:		
(Mrs. Paul's):		
Breaded & fried	½ of 7-oz. pkg.	24.1
With butter & cheese	7-oz. pkg.	11.0
(Van de Kamp's) country seasoned	½ of 7-oz. pkg.	19.0
SCHNAPPS, PEPPERMINT (DeKuyper)	1 fl. oz.	7.5
*SCOTCH BROTH (Campbell)	8-oz. serving	8.8
SCOTCH SOUR COCKTAIL:		
(National Distillers) *Duet*, 12½% alcohol	8 fl. oz.	25.6
(Party Tyme) 12½% alcohol	2 fl. oz.	5.7
SCREWDRIVER:		
Canned:		
(National Distillers) *Duet*, 12½% alcohol	8-fl.-oz. can	25.6
(Party Tyme) 12½% alcohol	2 fl. oz.	6.4
Dry mix (Bar-Tender's; Holland House)	1 serving	17.4

Food and Description	Measure or Quantity	Carbohydrates (grams)
SEAFOOD PLATTER, frozen (Mrs. Paul's) breaded & fried	½ of 9-oz. pkg.	28.5
SECOND NATURE (Avoset) egg substitute	3 T.	1.8
SEGO DIET FOOD:		
Bars	1 bar	12.0
Canned:		
Chocolate, milk chocolate, very chocolate malt	10-fl.-oz. can	39.0
Very butterscotch, very vanilla	10-fl.-oz. can	35.0
SERUTAN:		
Toasted granules	1 tsp.	1.3
Concentrated powder	1 tsp.	1.3
Fruit-flavored powder	1 tsp.	1.5
SESAME SEEDS (French's)	1 tsp.	.9
SHAD, CREOLE	4 oz.	1.8
SHAKE 'N BAKE:		
Regular:		
Chicken	2.4-oz. pkg.	43.0
Chicken, barbecue style	3¾-oz. pkg.	83.2
Chicken, crispy country milk	2.4-oz. pkg.	50.1
Chicken, Italian flavor	2.3-oz. pkg.	41.4
Fish	2-oz. pkg.	33.9
Hamburger	2-oz. pkg.	33.2
Pork	2.4-oz. pkg.	47.1
Pork & ribs, barbecue style	2.9-oz. pkg.	61.2
Plus homestyle gravy mix:		
Beef	3.1-oz. pkg.	51.4
Pork	3.7-oz. pkg.	67.4
SHERBET (Dean)	¼ pt.	30.6
SHERRY:		
Cocktail (Gold Seal)	3 fl. oz.	1.6
Cream:		
(Great Western) Solera	3 fl. oz.	12.2
(Taylor)	3 fl. oz.	13.2
Dry:		
(Italian Swiss Colony) Gold Medal	3 fl. oz.	1.7
(Williams & Humbert)	3 fl. oz.	4.5
Dry Sack (Williams & Humbert)	3 fl. oz.	4.5
SHREDDED WHEAT:		
(Nabisco)	¾-oz. biscuit	17.0
(Nabisco) Spoon Size	⅔ cup	23.0
(Quaker)	2 biscuits	22.0
SHRIMP:		
Canned:		
(Bumble Bee) solids & liq.	4½-oz. can	.9
(Icy Point; Pillar Rock; Snow Mist) cocktail	4½-oz. can	.8
Frozen (Mrs. Paul's) fried	½ of 6-oz. pkg.	16.8
SHRIMP CAKE (Mrs. Paul's) thins	2½-oz. cake	1.4

Food and Description	Measure or Quantity	Carbohydrates (grams)
SHRIMP COCKTAIL:		
(Sau-Sea)	4-oz. jar	20.6
(Sea Snack)	4-oz. jar	14.8
SHRIMP DINNER, frozen (Van de Kamp's)	10-oz. dinner	40.0
SHRIMP PUFF (Durkee)	1 piece	3.0
SHRIMP SOUP:		
*(Campbell) cream of	10-oz. serving	17.0
(Crosse & Blackwell) cream of	½ of 13-oz. can	7.0
(Snow) New England	15-oz. can	44.9
SHRIMP STICKS, frozen (Mrs. Paul's)	.8-oz. stick	5.5
SIDE CAR COCKTAIL MIX (Holland House)	2 fl. oz.	22.0
SLENDER (Carnation):		
Bar	1 bar	11.5
Dry	1 packet	20.0
Liquid	10-fl.-oz. can	34.0
SLIM JIM	1 piece	.4
SLOPPY JOE:		
Canned:		
(Libby's) beef	⅓ cup	6.0
(Libby's) pork	⅓ cup	5.7
(Morton House) beef	5-oz. serving	19.0
Frozen:		
(Banquet) cooking bag	5-oz. bag	11.2
(Green Giant) with tomato sauce & beef, *Toast Topper*	5-oz. pkg.	14.3
SLOPPY JOE SEASONING MIX:		
(Ann Page)	1½-oz. pkg.	28.8
*(Durkee)	¼ cup	6.0
(French's)	1½-oz. pkg.	32.0
SMOKIE SAUSAGE:		
(Hormel)	1 piece	.4
(Vienna)	2½-oz. serving	.9
SNO BALL (Hostess)	1 cake	25.1
SOAVE WINE (Antinori)	3 fl. oz.	6.3
SOFT DRINK:		
Sweetened:		
Apple (Shasta) red	6 fl. oz.	20.6
Birch beer:		
(Pennsylvania Dutch)	6 fl. oz.	19.7
(Yukon Club)	6 fl. oz.	22.3
Bitter lemon:		
(Canada Dry)	6 fl. oz.	19.2
(Schweppes)	6 fl. oz.	20.3
Bubble Up	6 fl. oz.	18.4
Cherry:		
(Canada Dry) wild	6 fl. oz.	24.0
(Cott)	6 fl. oz.	23.0
(Nedick's) black	6 fl. oz.	20.1
(Shasta) black	6 fl. oz.	21.8

Food and Description	Measure or Quantity	Carbohydrates (grams)
(Yoo-Hoo) high protein	6 fl. oz.	18.9
Chocolate:		
(Cott) cream	6 fl. oz.	22.0
(Yoo-Hoo) high protein	6 fl. oz.	18.9
Club Soda: (all brands)	6 fl. oz.	0
Cola:		
Coca-Cola	6 fl. oz.	18.0
(Cott)	6 fl. oz.	20.0
Jamaica (Canada Dry)	6 fl. oz.	19.8
(Mission)	6 fl. oz.	20.0
Mr. Cola	6 fl. oz.	20.3
Pepsi-Cola	6 fl. oz.	19.9
RC (Royal Crown) with a twist	6 fl. oz.	20.5
(Royal Crown)	6 fl. oz.	19.5
(Shasta) cherry	6 fl. oz.	19.8
Cream:		
(Canada Dry) vanilla	6 fl. oz.	24.0
(Cott)	6 fl. oz.	22.0
(Nedick's)	6 fl. oz.	20.9
(Shasta)	6 fl. oz.	20.6
Dr. Brown's Cel-Ray Tonic	6 fl. oz.	16.5
Dr. Pepper	6 fl. oz.	18.6
Ginger Ale:		
(Canada Dry)	6 fl. oz.	15.6
(Cott)	6 fl. oz.	15.0
(Schweppes)	6 fl. oz.	16.3
(Shasta)	6 fl. oz.	15.9
Ginger beer (Schweppes)	6 fl. oz.	16.8
Grape:		
(Canada Dry) concord	6 fl. oz.	24.0
(Fanta)	6 fl. oz.	21.8
(Hi-C)	6 fl. oz.	20.0
(Nedick's)	6 fl. oz.	23.2
(Patio)	6 fl. oz.	24.0
(Schweppes)	6 fl. oz.	15.7
Grapefruit:		
(Cott)	6 fl. oz.	20.0
(Shasta)	6 fl. oz.	21.8
Half & Half (Kirsch)	6 fl. oz.	20.3
Hi Spot (Canada Dry)	6 fl. oz.	18.6
Lemon (Clicquot Club; Cott; Mission)	6 fl. oz.	18.0
Lemonade (Hi-C)	6 fl. oz.	20.0
Lemon-lime:		
(Dr. Brown's; Hoffman's; Key Food; Nedick's; Waldbaum; Yukon Club)	6 fl. oz.	18.4
(Shasta)	6 fl. oz.	19.1
Mello Yello	6 fl. oz.	22.5
Mountain Dew	6 fl. oz.	22.1
Mr. Pibb	6 fl. oz.	18.8

Food and Description	Measure or Quantity	Carbohydrates (grams)
Orange:		
(Canada Dry) *Sunripe*	6 fl. oz.	14.1
(Clicquot Club; Cott; Mission)	6 fl. oz.	25.0
(Fanta)	6 fl. oz.	22.5
(Hi-C)	6 fl. oz.	20.0
(Shasta)	6 fl. oz.	23.9
Quinine or Tonic Water:		
(Canada Dry)	6 fl. oz.	16.1
(Schweppes)	6 fl. oz.	16.5
(Shasta)	6 fl. oz.	16.1
Raspberry:		
(Clicquot Club; Cott; Mission)	6 fl. oz.	24.0
(Shasta) wild	6 fl. oz.	21.8
Red creme (Schweppes)	6 fl. oz.	21.3
Rondo (Schweppes)	6 fl. oz.	19.6
Root beer:		
Barrelhead (Canada Dry)	6 fl. oz.	19.8
(Cott)	6 fl. oz.	21.0
(Dad's)	6 fl. oz.	19.6
(Fanta)	6 fl. oz.	20.3
(Hires)	6 fl. oz.	18.8
(Patio)	6 fl. oz.	20.8
Rooti (Canada Dry)	6 fl. oz.	19.8
(Schweppes)	6 fl. oz.	19.3
(Shasta) draft	6 fl. oz.	20.5
Sarsaparilla (Hoffman)	6 fl. oz.	22.2
Seven-Up	6 fl. oz.	18.0
Sprite	6 fl. oz.	18.0
Strawberry:		
(Canada Dry) California	6 fl. oz.	22.3
(Salute)	6 fl. oz.	24.3
(Shasta)	6 fl. oz.	21.8
Tahitian Treat (Canada Dry)	6 fl. oz.	24.1
Teem	6 fl. oz.	17.7
Tiki (Shasta)	6 fl. oz.	20.6
Tom Collins or Collins Mix:		
(Canada Dry; Yukon Club)	6 fl. oz.	15.0
(Shasta)	6 fl. oz.	16.1
Vanilla cream (Canada Dry)	6 fl. oz.	22.0
Wink (Canada Dry)	6 fl. oz.	22.7
Dietetic or low calorie:		
Apple (Shasta) red	6 fl. oz.	.2
Bubble Up	6 fl. oz.	.2
Cherry:		
(Clicquot Club; Cott; Mission)	6 fl. oz.	.3
(No-Cal; Shasta)	6 fl. oz.	0
(Tab) black	6 fl. oz.	Tr.
Chocolate:		
(Hoffman)	6 fl. oz.	.2
(No-Cal)	6 fl. oz.	<.1
(Shasta)	6 fl. oz.	0
Chocolate Mint (No-Cal)	6 fl. oz.	<.1

Food and Description	Measure or Quantity	Carbohydrates (grams)
Coffee:		
(Hoffman)	6 fl. oz.	.8
(No-Cal)	6 fl. oz.	.3
Cola:		
(Canada Dry)	6 fl. oz.	.6
(Clicquot Club; Cott; Mission)	6 fl. oz.	.1
Diet Rite	6 fl. oz.	Tr.
(No-Cal)	6 fl. oz.	<.1
Pepsi, diet	6 fl. oz.	<.1
Pepsi Light	6 fl. oz.	6.4
RC	6 fl. oz.	Tr.
(Shasta) regular & cherry	6 fl. oz.	0
(Yukon Club)	6 fl. oz.	.3
Tab	6 fl. oz.	<.1
Cream:		
(Dr. Brown's; Hoffman; Key Food; Waldbaum; Yukon Club)	6 fl. oz.	.2
(No-Cal)	6 fl. oz.	<.1
(Shasta)	6 fl. oz.	0
Dr. Pepper	6 fl. oz.	.4
Fresca	6 fl. oz.	0
Ginger Ale:		
(Canada Dry)	6 fl. oz.	0
(Dr. Brown's; Hoffman; Key Food; Waldbaum) pale dry	6 fl. oz.	.2
(No-Cal)	6 fl. oz.	Tr.
(Shasta)	6 fl. oz.	0
Tab	6 fl. oz.	Tr.
Grape:		
(No-Cal; Shasta)	6 fl. oz.	0
Tab	6 fl. oz.	0
Grapefruit:		
(Hoffman)	6 fl. oz.	.4
(Shasta)	6 fl. oz.	.3
Lemon (Clicquot Club; Cott; Mission)	6 fl. oz.	.5
Lemon-Lime:		
Diet Rite	6 fl. oz.	.4
(Shasta)	6 fl. oz.	0
Tab	6 fl. oz.	0
Mr. Pipp	6 fl. oz.	0
Orange:		
(*Diet Rite*; Dr. Brown's; Hoffman; Key Food; Waldbaum)	6 fl. oz.	.2
(Nedick's; Yukon Club)	6 fl. oz.	.4
(No-Cal; Shasta)	6 fl. oz.	0
Tab	6 fl. oz.	0
Quinine or tonic water (No-Cal; Shasta)	6 fl. oz.	0

Food and Description	Measure or Quantity	Carbohydrates (grams)
Raspberry:		
(Dr. Brown's; Hoffman; Key Food; Waldbaum) black	6 fl. oz.	.4
(No-Cal) black	6 fl. oz.	<.1
(Shasta) wild	6 fl. oz.	0
Red Pop (No-Cal)	6 fl. oz.	0
Root Beer:		
Barrelhead (Canada Dry)	6 fl. oz.	.8
(Dad's; Hoffman)	6 fl. oz.	.2
(No-Cal)	6 fl. oz.	Tr.
(Shasta) draft	6 fl. oz.	0
Tab	6 fl. oz.	<.1
Seven-Up	6 fl. oz.	.6
Shape-Up (No-Cal)	6 fl. oz.	0
Sprite	6 fl. oz.	0
Strawberry:		
(Clicquot Club; Cott; Mission)	6 fl. oz.	.5
(Shasta)	6 fl. oz.	0
Tab	6 fl. oz.	0
Tea (No-Cal)	6 fl. oz.	0
Tiki (Shasta)	6 fl. oz.	0
TNT (No-Cal)	6 fl. oz.	0
SOLE, frozen:		
(Mrs. Paul's) fillets, breaded & fried	4-oz. serving	21.8
(Mrs. Paul's) fillets, with lemon butter	4½-oz. serving	9.7
(Van de Kamp's) batter dipped, french fried	1 piece	12.0
(Weight Watchers)	16-oz. meal	14.1
SOUTHERN COMFORT:		
86 proof	1 fl. oz.	3.5
100 proof	1 fl. oz.	3.5
SOYBEAN CURD or **TOFU**	2¾" x 1½" x 1" cake	2.9
SOYBEAN or **NUT:**		
Dry roasted (*Soy Ahoy; Soy Town*)	1 oz.	6.0
Oil roasted (*Soy Ahoy; Soy Town*) plain, barbecue or garlic	1 oz.	4.8
SPAGHETTI, cooked:		
8-10 minutes, *"al dente"*	1 cup	43.9
14-20 minutes, tender	1 cup	32.2
SPAGHETTI DINNER, frozen:		
(Banquet)	11½-oz. dinner	62.9
(Morton) & meatball	11-oz. dinner	59.4
(Swanson) *Hungry Man*	18½-oz. dinner	83.0
SPAGHETTI & FRANKFURTERS, canned		
(Franco-American) in tomato sauce, *SpaghettiOs*	½ of 14¾-oz. can	26.0
SPAGHETTI & MEATBALLS IN TOMATO SAUCE:		
Canned:		
(Franco-American)	7¼-oz. can	23.0

Food and Description	Measure or Quantity	Carbohydrates (grams)
(Franco-American) *SpaghettiOs*	½ of 14¾-oz. can	24.0
(Libby's)	7½-oz. can	27.5
Dietetic, canned (Dia-Mel) in sauce	8-oz. can	24.0
Dietetic, canned (Featherweight)	8-oz. can	28.0
Frozen (Banquet)	¼ of 32-oz. pkg.	32.3
Frozen (Green Giant) in tomato sauce	8-oz. entree	29.1
SPAGHETTI WITH MEAT SAUCE, frozen (Banquet)	8-oz. cooking bag	31.3
SPAGHETTI SAUCE:		
Clam, white (Buitoni)	5 oz.	2.2
Marinara (Ann Page)	¼ of 15½-oz. jar	12.3
Marinara (Prince)	4-oz. serving	12.4
Meat:		
(Buitoni)	5 oz.	5.0
(Prince)	½ cup	11.0
(Ragu) thick & zesty	5-oz. serving	14.0
(Ronzoni)	4 oz.	11.0
Meatless or plain:		
(Ann Page) meatless with mushrooms	¼ of 15½-oz. jar	12.5
(Prince)	½ cup	11.4
(Ragu)	5 oz.	14.0
(Ragu) extra thick & zesty	5 oz.	13.0
Mushroom:		
(Prince)	4 oz.	11.3
(Ragu)	5 oz.	13.0
Pepperoni (Ragu)	5 oz.	14.0
Dietetic (Featherweight) low sodium	5 oz.	10.0
SPAGHETTI SAUCE MIX:		
(Ann Page) with mushrooms	¼ pkg.	6.8
*(Durkee)	2½ cups	52.0
*(Durkee) mushroom	2⅔ cups	48.0
(French's) Italian style	1½-oz. pkg.	26.8
(Lawry's) with mushrooms	1½-oz. pkg.	22.6
*(Spatini)	2 oz. serving	4.0
SPAM (Hormel)	1 oz.	1.1
SPECIAL K, cereal (Kelloggs')	1¼ cups	21.0
SPINACH:		
Fresh, whole leaves	½ cup	.7
Boiled	½ cup	2.8
Canned (Libby's) solids & liq.	½ cup	3.6
Canned, dietetic (Featherweight) solids & liq.	½ cup	4.0
Frozen:		
(Birds Eye) chopped or leaf	⅓ pkg.	2.7
(Birds Eye) creamed	⅓ pkg.	4.0
(Green Giant):		
In butter sauce	⅓ pkg.	2.3

102

Food and Description	Measure or Quantity	Carbohydrates (grams)
Creamed	⅓ pkg.	7.8
Souffle	½ pkg.	8.2
SPINACH PUREE, dietetic (Cellu) low sodium	½ cup	3.5
SQUASH PUREE, dietetic (Cellu) low sodium	½ cup	9.5
SQUASH, SUMMER:		
Yellow, boiled, slices	½ cup	2.7
Zucchini, boiled, slices	½ cup	1.9
Canned (Del Monte) zucchini in tomato sauce	½ cup	7.9
SQUASH, WINTER:		
Acorn, baked	½ cup	14.3
Hubbard, baked, mashed	½ cup	11.9
Frozen (Birds Eye)	⅓ pkg.	11.0
SQUOZE (Pillsbury)	6 fl. oz.	10.0
START	½ cup	12.7
STRAWBERRY:		
Fresh, capped	½ cup	6.1
Frozen (Birds Eye):		
Halves	⅓ pkg.	48.2
Whole	¼ pkg.	23.2
Whole, quick thaw	½ pkg.	29.7
STRAWBERRY DRINK (Hi-C)	6 fl. oz.	22.0
STRAWBERRY ICE CREAM:		
(Meadow Gold) 10% fat	¼ pt.	16.0
(Swift)	½ cup	15.3
STRAWBERRY JELLY:		
Sweetened (Smucker's)	1 T.	13.5
Dietetic (Featherweight)	1 T.	4.0
STRAWBERRY PRESERVE:		
Sweetened (Bama; Smucker's)	1 T.	13.5
Dietetic or low calorie:		
(Dia-Mel; Louis Sherry)	1 tsp.	0
(Diet Delight; Featherweight)	1 T.	3.3
(Tillie Lewis)	1 tsp.	1.0
STRAWBERRY SYRUP:		
Sweetened (Smucker's)	1 T.	11.6
Dietetic (Featherweight)	1 T.	3.0
STUFFING MIX:		
*Chicken, *Stove Top*	½ cup	20.0
*Cornbread, *Stove Top*	½ cup	20.0
*Pork, *Stove Top*	½ cup	20.0
White bread, *Mrs. Cubbison's*	1 oz.	20.5
STURGEON, smoked	4 oz.	0
SUCCOTASH:		
Canned:		
(Libby's) cream style	½ cup	22.8
(Libby's) whole kernel	½ cup	16.0
(Stokely Van Camp)	½ cup	17.5
Frozen (Birds Eye)	⅓ pkg.	17.0

Food and Description	Measure or Quantity	Carbohydrates (grams)
SUGAR:		
Brown	1 T.	12.5
Confectioners'	1 T.	7.7
Granulated	1 T.	11.9
Maple	1¾" x 1¼" x ½" piece	27.0
SUGAR CORN POPS, cereal	1 cup	26.0
SUGAR CRISP, cereal	⅞ cup	25.5
SUGAR FROSTED FLAKES, cereal:		
(Kellogg's)	⅔ cup	26.0
(Ralston Purina)	¾ cup	26.0
SUGAR SMACKS, cereal	¾ cup	25.0
SUGAR SUBSTITUTE:		
Sprinkle Sweet (Pillsbury)	1 tsp.	.5
Sugar-Like (Dia-Mel)	1 packet	1.0
Sug'r Like (Featherweight)	1 tsp.	1.0
Sweet'n-it (Dia-Mel) liquid	5 drops	0
SUNDAE, canned, *Swiss Miss:*		
Chocolate	4½ oz.	28.0
Vanilla	4½ oz.	26.0
SUNFLOWER SEED:		
In hulls	1 oz.	3.1
Hulled (Planters)	1 oz.	5.4
Dry roasted (Planters)	1 oz.	4.0
SUNNY DOODLES (Drake's)	1 cake	17.1
SUZY Q (Hostess):		
Banana	1 cake	38.4
Chocolate	1 cake	36.5
SWEETBREADS, calf, braised	4 oz.	0
SWEET POTATO:		
Baked, peeled	5" x 1" sweet potato	35.8
Canned, heavy syrup	4 oz.	31.2
Frozen:		
(Green Giant) glazed	⅓ pkg.	22.7
(Mrs. Paul's) candied, with apple	4-oz. serving	37.2
SWEET & SOUR ORIENTAL, canned (La Choy):		
Chicken	8½-oz. serving	71.1
Pork	8½-oz. serving	69.0
SWISS ROLL (Drake's)	1 roll	47.4
SWISS STEAK (Swanson)	10-oz. dinner	19.0
SWORDFISH, broiled	3" x 3" x ½" steak	0

T

TABASCO	¼ tsp.	<.1
TACO:		
*(Ortega)	1 taco	13.0
(Patio) cocktail	½-oz. taco	4.8
*Mix (Durkee)	½ cup	3.8
TAMALE, canned (Derby)	1 tamale	6.5

Food and Description	Measure or Quantity	Carbohydrates (grams)
*TANG, grape or orange	½ cup	15.0
TANGERINE or MANDARIN ORANGE:		
Fresh (Sunkist)	1 large tangerine	10.0
Canned (Diet Delight)	½ cup	11.7
*TANGERINE JUICE, frozen (Minute Maid)	6 fl. oz.	20.8
TARRAGON (French's)	1 tsp.	.7
TEA:		
(Lipton)	1 bag	0
(Tender Leaf)	1 rounded tsp.	0
Canned, (Lipton) lemon flavor	12-fl.-oz. can	32.0
Iced (See TEA MIX, iced)		
TEAM, cereal	1 cup	24.0
TEA, MIX, iced:		
*(Lipton) lemon-flavored	1 cup	16.0
*Nestea, lemon-flavored	8 fl. oz.	.2
TEMPTYS (Tastykake) butter creme, chocolate or lemon	¾-oz. cake	12.9
TEXTURED VEGETABLE PROTEIN:		
Breakfast link, *Morningstar Farms*	1 link	.3
Breakfast patties, *Morningstar Farms*	1 pattie	3.1
Breakfast strips, *Morningstar Farms*	1 strip	.2
Grillers, *Morningstar Farms*	1 patty	5.3
Hamburger (Williams)	4-oz. pkg.	53.6
Luncheon slices, *Morningstar Farms*	1 slice	1.4
Meatloaf (Williams)	4-oz. pkg.	54.2
*Pathmark	4 oz.	2.9
THUNDERBIRD WINE (Gallo):		
14% alcohol	3 fl. oz.	8.1
20% alcohol	3 fl. oz.	7.5
THURINGER, beef (Oscar Mayer)	.8-oz. slice	.5
THYME LEAVES (French's)	1 tsp.	1.0
TIA MARIA, liqueur (Hiram Walker)	1 fl. oz.	10.0
TIGER TAILS (Hostess)	1 piece	76.2
TOASTER CAKE:		
(Nabisco) all varieties	1 piece	35.0
(Thomas'):		
Blueberry	1 piece	17.5
Bran	1 piece	19.6
Corn	1 piece	18.3
TOASTER SANDWICH (Borden):		
Cheese zesty	1 sandwich	16.8
Grilled cheese	1 sandwich	16.6
Pizza	1 sandwich	17.0
TOASTY O's, cereal	1 oz.	19.9
TOFFEE KRUNCH BAR (Sealtest)	3 fl. oz.	12.0

Food and Description	Measure or Quantity	Carbohydrates (grams)
TOMATO:		
Cherry, whole	4 pieces	3.2
Regular, whole	1 med.	7.0
Canned, regular pack:		
(Contadina) sliced	4 oz.	8.5
(Stokely-Van Camp) stewed	½ cup	7.5
(Van Camp) whole	½ cup	5.0
Canned, dietetic (Featherweight)	½ cup	4.0
TOMATO & HOT GREEN CHILI PEPPERS, canned (Ortega)	1 oz.	1.4
TOMATO JUICE:		
(Campbell)	6-fl.-oz. can	8.0
(Del Monte)	6-fl.-oz. can	7.4
(Libby's)	6 fl. oz.	7.5
(Sacramento)	5½-fl.-oz. can	7.7
Dietetic (Diet Delight; Featherweight; Tillie Lewis)	6 fl. oz.	7.5
TOMATO JUICE COCKTAIL:		
(Sacramento) peppy	5½-fl.-oz. can	9.1
(Sacramento) *Tomato Plus*	5½-fl.-oz. can	9.9
Snap-E-Tom	6-fl.-oz. can	6.8
TOMATO PASTE:		
(Contadina)	6-oz. can	35.0
Dietetic (Featherweight)	6-oz. can	35.0
TOMATO PRESERVE (Smucker's)	1 T.	13.5
TOMATO PUREE:		
Canned (Contadina) heavy	1 cup	26.4
Canned, dietetic (Cellu)	1 cup	20.0
TOMATO SAUCE:		
(Contadina)	1 cup	19.6
(Del Monte)	1 cup	17.0
(Del Monte) with tomato tidbits	1 cup	5.7
(Hunt's) with cheese	4 oz.	10.0
(Hunt's) *Prima Salsa*, regular & mushroom	4 oz.	20.0
TOMATO SOUP:		
Canned:		
*(Ann Page)	1 cup	14.1
*(Ann Page) & rice	1 cup	20.1
*(Campbell)	10-oz. serving	27.0
*(Campbell) & beef, *Noodle-O's*	10-oz. serving	24.0
*(Campbell) bisque	10-oz. serving	27.0
*(Campbell) & rice	10-oz. serving	26.0
(Progresso)	1 cup	23.0
Dietetic:		
(Campbell) low sodium	7¼-oz. can	22.0
*(Dia-Mel)	8-oz. serving	11.0
*Mix (Nestlé's *Souptime*; Lipton *Cup-a-Soup*)	6 fl. oz.	13.0
TOM COLLINS:		
Canned (Party Tyme) 10% alcohol	2 fl. oz.	5.9
Mix, dry (Holland House)	1 serving	17.0

Food and Description	Measure or Quantity	Carbohydrates (grams)
Mix, dry (Party Tyme)	½-oz. pkg.	13.3
Mix, liquid (Holland House)	2 fl. oz.	30.0
TONGUE, beef, braised	4 oz.	.5
TONGUE, canned (Hormel)	1 oz.	<.1
TOPPING:		
Butterscotch (Kraft)	1 T.	12.4
Caramel (Kraft)	1 T.	16.7
Chocolate fudge (Hershey's)	1 T.	9.3
Chocolate fudge (Kraft)	1 T.	10.9
Marshmallow (Kraft)	1 T.	9.4
Pecan in syrup (Smucker's)	1 T.	14.0
Pineapple (Kraft)	1 oz.	19.7
Spoonmallow (Kraft)	1 oz.	21.9
Walnut (Kraft)	1 oz.	14.3
Dietetic, chocolate (Diet Delight)	1 T.	2.1
TOPPING, WHIPPED:		
(Birds Eye) Cool Whip	1 T.	1.3
(Lucky Whip)	1 T.	.5
(Rich's) WhipTopping	¼ oz.	1.2
Richwhip	1 T.	1.2
Frozen (Rich's) Spoon 'n Serve	1 T.	1.1
Mix:		
*(Dream Whip)	1 T.	1.0
*Dietetic (D-Zerta)	1 T.	0
TORTILLA (Amigos)	6" x ⅛" tortilla	19.7
TOTAL, cereal (General Mills)	1 cup	23.0
TRAMINER WINE (Inglenook)	3 fl. oz.	.5
TRIPE, canned (Libby's)	6-oz. serving	1.1
TRIPLE SEC LIQUEUR:		
(Bols)	1 fl. oz.	8.8
(DeKuyper)	1 fl. oz.	8.7
(Garnier)	1 fl. oz.	8.5
TRIX, cereal	1 cup	25.0
TROPICAL PUNCH DRINK (Wagner)	6 fl. oz.	25.2
TROUT, frozen dressed (1000 Springs)	5-oz. trout	3.2
TUNA:		
Canned in oil:		
(Breast o' Chicken) solids & liq.	6½-oz. can	0
(Bumble Bee) drained	½ cup	0
(Carnation) solids & liq.	6½-oz. can	0
(Chicken of the Sea) chunk light, solids & liq.	6½-oz. can	<1.8
(Star Kist) solid white, solids & liq.	7 oz.	0
Canned in water:		
(Breast o' Chicken)	6½-oz. can	0
(Star-Kist) light	7-oz. can	0
(Chicken of the Sea) white	7-oz. can	1.0
(Featherweight)	6½-oz. can	0

Food and Description	Measure or Quantity	Carbohydrates (grams)
TUNA HELPER (General Mills):		
Creamy noodle	⅕ pkg.	30.0
Creamy rice	⅕ pkg.	33.0
Macaroni newburg	⅕ pkg.	29.0
Noodles & cheese sauce	⅕ pkg.	28.0
TUNA & PEAS, frozen (Green Giant) creamed	5 oz.	9.8
TUNA PIE:		
(Banquet)	8-oz. pie	42.7
(Morton)	8-oz. pie	36.4
TUNA SALAD:		
Home recipe	4 oz.	4.0
Canned (Carnation)	1½ oz.	3.2
TURBOT MEAL, frozen:		
(Weight Watchers)	8-oz. meal	12.0
(Weight Watchers) stuffed	16-oz. meal	25.9
TURKEY:		
Canned (Swanson)	5-oz. can	0
Roasted:		
Flesh & skin	4 oz.	0
Dark meat	2½" x 1⅝" x ¼" slice	0
Light meat	4" x 2" x ¼" slice	0
TURKEY DINNER, frozen:		
(Banquet)	11-oz. dinner	27.8
(Banquet) *Man Pleaser*	19-oz. dinner	73.8
(Morton) sliced, *Country Table*	15-oz. dinner	89.5
(Swanson)	11½-oz. dinner	45.0
(Swanson) *Hungry Man*	19-oz. dinner	80.0
(Swanson) 3-course	16-oz. dinner	60.0
(Weight Watchers) sliced	16-oz. meal	26.8
TURKEY PIE:		
(Banquet)	8-oz. pie	40.6
(Morton)	8-oz. pie	31.8
(Swanson)	8-oz. pie	40.0
(Swanson) *Hungry Man*	1-lb. pie	60.0
TURKEY SOUP:		
*(Ann Page) & noodle	1 cup	17.8
*(Ann Page) & vegetable	1 cup	8.9
(Campbell) *Chunky*	18½-oz. can	34.0
*(Campbell) & noodle	10-oz.	10.0
Dietetic (Campbell) low sodium, & noodle	7½-oz. can	14.0
TURMERIC (French's)	1 tsp.	1.3
TWINKIE (Hostess):		
Regular	1 cake	26.1
Devil's food	1 cake	24.7

V

VALPOLICELLA WINE (Antinori)	3 fl. oz.	6.3
VANDERMINT, liqueur	1 fl. oz.	10.2

Food and Description	Measure or Quantity	Carbohydrates (grams)
VANILLA EXTRACT (Virginia Dare)	1 tsp.	Tr.
VANILLA ICE CREAM:		
(Borden):		
10.5% fat	¼ pt.	15.8
Lady Borden	¼ pt.	17.0
(Breyer's) & strawberry	¼ pt.	20.0
(Dean) 10.1% fat	1 cup	33.8
(Meadow Gold) 10% fat	¼ pt.	15.0
(Prestige) French	¼ pt.	15.8
(Sealtest):		
Party Slice	¼ pt.	16.0
10.2% fat	¼ pt.	16.0
Fudge royale	¼ pt.	20.0
(Swift)	½ cup	15.7
VANILLA ICE MILK (Borden)		
Lite Line	¼ pt.	17.2
VEAL, broiled, medium-cooked:		
Loin, chop	4 oz.	0
Rib, roasted	4 oz.	0
Steak or cutlet, lean & fat	4 oz.	0
VEAL DINNER, frozen:		
(Banquet) parmigiana	11-oz. dinner	42.1
(Green Giant) parmigiana	7-oz. serving	18.3
(Morton) parmigiana	10¼-oz. dinner	46.6
(Swanson) parmigiana	12¼-oz. dinner	41.0
(Swanson) parmigiana, *Hungry Man*	20½-oz. dinner	70.0
V-8 (Campbell)	6-fl.-oz. can	8.0
VEGETABLES, MIXED:		
Canned:		
(Chun King) chow mein, solids & liq.	8-oz. serving	7.3
(Del Monte) drained solids	½ cup	7.4
(La Choy) chinese	1 cup	1.6
(La Choy) chop suey	1 cup	6.9
(Libby's) solids & liq.	½ cup	9.8
(Stokely-Van Camp) solids & liq.	½ cup	8.5
(Veg-All)	½ cup	7.8
Dietetic (Featherweight) low sodium	½ cup	8.0
Frozen:		
(Birds Eye):		
American Recipe:		
New England style	⅓ pkg.	11.7
New Orleans style	⅓ pkg.	13.8
Pennsylvania Dutch style	⅓ pkg.	7.3
San Francisco style	⅓ pkg.	6.4
Wisconsin style	⅓ pkg.	6.4
International:		
Bavarian style	⅓ pkg.	10.6

Food and Description	Measure or Quantity	Carbohydrates (grams)
Chinese style	⅓ pkg.	10.2
Hawaiian style	⅓ pkg.	12.0
Italian style	⅓ pkg.	8.3
Japanese style	⅓ pkg.	9.1
Stir Fry:		
Chinese style	⅓ pkg.	7.0
Mandarin style	⅓ pkg.	6.0
(Green Giant):		
Chinese style	½ cup	10.0
Hawaiian style	½ cup	16.5
Mixed	½ cup	8.0
(Kounty Kist)	½ cup	8.0
(La Choy) Chinese	5-oz. serving	5.3
(La Choy) Japanese	5-oz. serving	5.8
(Ore-Ida) stew vegetables	⅛ of 24-oz. pkg.	13.0
VEGETABLE SOUP:		
Canned:		
*(Ann Page):		
Beef stock	1 cup	20.0
Vegetarian	1 cup	12.3
(Campbell):		
*Regular	10 oz.	17.0
*Beef	10 oz.	10.0
Chunky	10¾-oz. can	25.0
Old World, *Soup For One*	7¾-oz. can	18.0
*Vegetarian	10 oz.	16.0
Dietetic:		
(Campbell) low sodium	7¼-oz. can	15.0
*(Dia-Mel)	8 oz.	12.0
*Mix (Lipton):		
Alphabet, *Cup-a-Soup*	1 pkg.	6.0
Beef	1 cup	9.0
Beef with shells	1 cup	18.0
Italian vegetable	1 cup	19.0
VEGETARIAN FOODS:		
Canned or dry:		
Big franks, drained (Loma Linda)	1.9-oz. frank	4.0
Chili (Worthington)	¼ can (5 oz.)	20.0
Chili beans (Loma Linda)	½ cup	21.1
Choplet (Worthington)	1 choplet	3.0
Cutlet (Worthington)	1 cutlet	2.6
Dinner cuts, drained (Loma Linda)	1 cut	1.6
FriChik (Worthington)	1 piece	1.0
Granburger (Worthington)	6 T.	12.0
Gravy Quik:		
Brown (Loma Linda)	.7-oz. packet	11.0
Mushroom (Loma Linda)	.7-oz. packet	11.5
Linketts, drained (Loma Linda)	1.3-oz. link	4.1
Nuteena (Loma Linda)	½" slice	7.5
Proteena (Loma Linda)	½" slice	6.5

Food and Description	Measure or Quantity	Carbohydrates (grams)
Protose (Worthington)	½" slice	7.0
Sandwich spread (Loma Linda)	1 T.	1.7
Saucette (Worthington)	1.2-oz. link	1.5
Soyagen, all-purpose powder (Loma Linda)	1 T.	4.7
Soyalac (Loma Linda):		
I-soyalac	1 cup	33.8
Concentrate, liquid	1 cup	33.8
Powder	1 cup	63.1
Ready to use	1 cup	16.1
Soyameat (Worthington):		
Sliced beef	1 slice	1.5
Diced chicken	¼ cup	2.0
Sliced chicken	1 slice	1.0
Salisbury steak	1 slice	2.0
Soyamel, any kind (Worthington)	1 oz.	15.2
Spaghetti sauce (Loma Linda)	½ cup	63.1
Super links (Worthington)	1 link	4.0
Tender bits, drained (Loma Linda)	1 piece	2.2
Tender rounds, drained (Loma Linda)	1 round	2.6
Vegeburger (Loma Linda)	½ cup	4.4
Vegeburger, no salt added (Loma Linda)	½ cup	7.0
Vegelona (Loma Linda)	½" slice	6.9
Vegetarian burger (Worthington)	⅓ cup	6.0
Vega-Links (Worthington)	1 link	1.5
Wheat protein	4 oz.	10.0
Wheat protein, nuts or peanuts	4 oz.	20.1
Wheat & soy protein	4 oz.	8.6
Wheat & soy protein, soy or other vegetable oil	4 oz.	10.8
Worthington 209	1 slice	1.5
Frozen:		
Beef-like roll (Worthington)	2½-oz. piece	4.0
Beef pie (Worthington)	1 pie	51.0
Bologna (Loma Linda)	1 oz.	2.8
Breakfast links (Loma Linda)	.7-oz. link	1.4
Breakfast sausage (Loma Linda)	1 oz.	1.4
Burger patties (Loma Linda)	3-oz. patty	11.4
Chicken (Loma Linda)	1 slice	1.5
Chicken pie (Worthington)	1 pie	42.0
Chic-Ketts (Worthington)	½ cup	6.0
Croquettes (Worthington)	1 croquette	5.0
FriPats (Worthington)	1 pat	3.0
Meatballs (Loma Linda)	1 meatball	2.2
Prosage (Worthington)	1 link	1.7
Roast beef (Loma Linda)	½" slice	3.8
Sizzle Burger (Loma Linda)	1 burger	10.0
Smoked beef, roll (Worthington)	2½ oz.	7.0
Stripples (Worthington)	1 slice	.8

Food and Description	Measure or Quantity	Carbohydrates (grams)
Turkey (Loma Linda)	½" slice	4.8
Wham (Worthington) roll	2½ oz.	4.0
VERMOUTH:		
Dry & extra dry (Lejon; Noilly Pratt)	1 fl. oz.	1.1
Sweet:		
(Lejon; Taylor)	1 fl. oz.	3.8
(Noilly Pratt)	1 fl. oz.	4.0
VICHYSSOISE SOUP (Crosse & Blackwell) cream of	½ of 13-oz. can	5.0
VIENNA SAUSAGE:		
(Armour Star)	.6-oz. sausage	0
(Libby's)	.7-oz. sausage	.5
(Wilson)	1 oz.	<.1
VINEGAR:	1 T.	.9
VIN KAFE (Lejon)	3 fl. oz.	22.8
VIRGIN SOUR MIX (Party Tyme)	½-oz. pkg.	13.3
VODKA & TONIC, canned (Party Tyme) 10% alcohol	2 fl. oz.	5.1

W

WAFFLE, frozen:		
(Aunt Jemima) jumbo	1 waffle	13.6
(Downyflake) jumbo	1 waffle	18.0
(Eggo):		
Blueberry	1 waffle	18.0
Bran	1 waffle	20.0
Plain	1 waffle	17.0
Strawberry	1 waffle	18.0
WALNUT, English or Persian (Diamond)	1 cup	12.8
WATER CHESTNUT, canned:		
(Chun King) drained	8½-oz. can	27.0
(La Choy) drained	8-oz. can	14.6
WATERCRESS	½ cup	.5
WATERMELON:		
Wedge	4" x 8" wedge	27.3
Diced	½ cup	5.1
WELSH RAREBIT:		
Home recipe	1 cup	14.6
Frozen (Green Giant)	5 oz.	11.4
WESTERN DINNER, frozen:		
(Banquet)	11-oz. dinner	32.4
(Morton) *Round-Up*	11¾-oz. dinner	33.4
(Swanson) *Hungry Man*	17¾-oz. dinner	77.0
WHEAT CHEX, cereal	⅔ cup	23.0
WHEATENA, cereal	¼ cup	23.0
WHEAT GERM CEREAL:		
(Kellogg's) plain	¼ cup	13.0
(Kellogg's) sugar & honey	¼ cup	17.0

Food and Description	Measure or Quantity	Carbohydrates (grams)
(Kretschmer) plain	¼ cup	13.0
(Kretschmer) sugar & honey	¼ cup	17.0
WHEATIES, cereal	1 cup	23.0
WHISKEY SOUR:		
(Hiram Walker)	3 fl. oz.	12.0
(National Distillers) *Duet*, 12½% alcohol	8-fl.-oz. can	17.6
Dry mix (Bar-Tender's)	1 serving	17.2
Dry mix (Holland House)	1 serving	17.0
Liquid mix (Holland House)	2 fl. oz.	26.0
WHITEFISH, LAKE:		
Baked, stuffed	4 oz.	6.6
Smoked	4 oz.	0
WILD BERRY DRINK (Hi-C)	6 fl. oz.	22.0
WILD RICE (Gourmet House)	⅓ cup	16.0
WINE, COOKING (Regina):		
Sauterne	¼ cup	.5
Sherry	¼ cup	4.7
WON TON SOUP:		
Canned (Mow Sang)	10-oz. can	21.0
*Frozen (La Choy)	1 cup	12.3

Y

YANKEE DOODLES (Drake's)	1 cake	15.6
YEAST, BAKER'S (Fleischmann's):		
Dry, active	¼ oz.	3.0
Fresh & household, active	.6-oz. cake	2.0
YOGURT:		
Regular:		
Plain:		
(Dannon)	8-oz. container	17.0
(Sealtest) *Light 'n Lively*	1 cup	18.0
Apple cinnamon (Breakstone)	8-oz. container	39.9
Apple crisp (New Country)	8-oz. container	41.4
Apricot:		
(Breakstone)	8-oz. container	37.4
(Breyer's)	1 cup	47.0
(Dannon)	8-oz. container	49.0
(Sealtest) *Light 'n Lively*	1 cup	48.0
Banana:		
(Breyer's)	1 cup	47.0
(Dannon)	8-oz. container	49.0
Blueberry:		
(Axelrod)	8-oz. container	41.0
(Breakstone)	8-oz. container	46.3
(Dannon)	8-oz. container	49.0
(Dean)	8-oz. container	50.6
(Meadow Gold) Swiss style	8-oz. container	49.0
(Sealtest) *Light 'n Lively*	1 cup	49.0
(Sweet 'n Low)	8-oz. container	28.0

Food and Description	Measure or Quantity	Carbohydrates (grams)
Blueberry ripple (New Country)	8-oz. container	43.0
Boysenberry:		
(Dannon)	8-oz. container	49.0
(Meadow Gold)	8-oz. container	54.0
Cherry:		
(Dannon)	8-oz. container	49.0
(Sweet 'n Low)	8-oz. container	28.0
Cherry supreme (New Country)	8-oz. container	44.0
Coffee (Dannon)	8-oz. container	32.0
Dutch apple (Dannon)	8-oz. container	49.0
Flavored, *Maya* (Alta-Dena)	1 container	39.0
Flavored, *Naja* (Alta-Dena)	1 container	40.0
French vanilla ripple (New Country)	8-oz. container	42.0
Fruit crunch (New Country)	8-oz. container	42.0
Grape (Breyer's)	1 cup	47.0
Hawaiian salad (New Country)	8-oz. container	42.0
Honey (Dannon)	8-oz. container	49.0
Honey'n Berries (New Country)	8-oz. container	43.0
Lemon:		
(Dannon)	8-oz. container	32.0
(Sealtest) *Light 'n Lively*	8-oz. container	47.0
(Sweet 'n Low)	8-oz. container	28.0
Lemon ripple (New Country)	8-oz. container	43.0
Mandarin orange (Borden) Swiss style	8-oz. container	45.9
Orange (Dean)	8-oz. container	62.9
Orange supreme (New Country)	8-oz. container	43.0
Peach:		
(Borden) Swiss style	8-oz. container	44.5
(Dannon)	8-oz. container	49.0
(Dean)	8-oz. container	49.1
(Sealtest) *Light 'n Lively*	8-oz. container	48.0
(Sweet 'n Low)	8-oz. container	28.0
Peach melba (Sealtest) *Light 'n Lively*	8-oz. container	48.0
Peaches 'n Cream (New Country)	8-oz. container	43.0
Pineapple:		
(Breakstone)	8-oz. container	37.9
(Breyer's)	8-oz. container	47.0
(Meadow Gold)	8-oz. container	54.0
(Sealtest) *Light 'n Lively*	8-oz. container	50.0
Pineapple-orange (Dannon)	8-oz. container	49.0
Raspberry:		
(Breakstone)	8-oz. container	45.8
(Breyer's) red	1 cup	47.0
(Dannon) red	8-oz. container	49.0
(Dean) red	8-oz. container	53.6
(Meadow Gold) Swiss style	8-oz. container	49.0
(Sealtest) *Light 'n Lively*	8-oz. container	43.0
(Sweet 'n Low)	8-oz. container	28.0
Raspberry ripple (New Country)	8-oz. container	43.0

Food and Description	Measure or Quantity	Carbohydrates (grams)
Strawberry:		
(Axelrod)	8-oz. container	40.6
(Breakstone)	8-oz. container	43.5
(Dannon)	8-oz. container	49.0
(Dean)	8-oz. container	46.8
(Meadow Gold)	8-oz. container	54.0
(Meadow Gold) Swiss style	8-oz. container	49.0
(Sealtest) *Light 'n Lively*	8-oz. container	47.0
(Sweet 'n Low)	8-oz. container	28.0
Strawberry supreme (New Country)	8-oz. container	43.0
Vanilla:		
(Breakstone)	8-oz. container	29.5
(Dannon)	8-oz. container	32.0
Frozen (Dannon):		
Banana:		
Danno-Yo	3½-oz. serving	21.0
Danny-in-a-Cup	8-oz. cup	42.0
Blueberry, *Danny Parfait*	4-oz. serving	35.0
Boysenberry:		
Danny-On-A-Stick, carob coated	2½-fl.-oz. bar	13.0
Danny-Yo	3½-oz. serving	21.0
Cherry, *Danny-in-a-Cup*	1 cup	42.0
Chocolate, *Danny-Yo*	3½-oz. serving	21.0
Lemon, *Danny-in-a-Cup*	8-oz. cup	20.0
Peach:		
Danny-in-a-Cup	8-oz. cup	42.0
Danny Parfait	4-oz. serving	35.0
Pina Colada:		
Danny-in-a-Cup	8-oz. cup	42.0
Danny-On-A-Stick	2½-fl.-oz. bar	13.0
Pineapple-orange, *Danny Parfait*	4-oz. serving	35.0
Raspberry, red:		
Danny-On-A-Stick, chocolate coated	2½-fl.-oz. bar	13.0
Danny-in-a-Cup	8-oz. container	42.0
Danny Parfait	4-oz. serving	35.0
Strawberry:		
Danny-in-a-Cup	8-oz. cup	42.0
Danny Flip, with strawberry topping	5-fl.-oz. serving	37.0
Danny Parfait	4-oz. serving	35.0
Danny-On-A-Stick	2½-fl.-oz. bar	13.0
Danny-On-A-Stick, chocolate coated	2½-fl.-oz. bar	13.0
Danny Yo	3½-oz. serving	21.0
Vanilla:		
Danny-in-a-Cup	8-oz. cup	20.0
Danny Flip, with red raspberry topping	5 fl. oz.	37.0

Food and Description	Measure or Quantity	Carbohydrates (grams)
Danny-On-A-Stick	2½-fl.-oz. bar	13.0
Danny-On-A-Stick, carob coated	2½-fl.-oz. bar	13.0
Danny Yo	3½-oz. serving	21.0
Vanilla-strawberry, *Danny Sampler*	3-fl.-oz. serving	14.0
YOGURT CHIFFON PIE, frozen (Sara Lee) *Light 'n Luscious:*		
Blueberry	⅛ of pie	20.4
Cherry	⅛ of pie	21.1
Strawberry	⅛ of pie	19.4
YOGURT DRINK MIX, *Sippin'* Yogurt (Alba):		
Orange, raspberry or strawberry flavor	1½-oz. envelope	31.0
Plain or Fancy	.8-oz. envelope	11.0

Z

ZINFANDEL WINE:		
(Inglenook) Vintage	3 fl. oz.	.3
(Italian Swiss Colony)	3 fl. oz.	.9
ZITI, frozen (Ronzoni)	4½ oz.	19.0
ZWIEBACK (Nabisco)	1 piece	5.0